Cardiothoracic Surgical Procedures and Techniques

J. Ernesto Molina

Cardiothoracic Surgical Procedures and Techniques

A Practical Manual

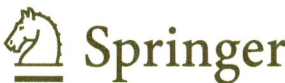 Springer

J. Ernesto Molina
Division of Cardiothoracic Surgery
University of Minnesota
Minneapolis, MN
USA

ISBN 978-3-030-09350-1   ISBN 978-3-319-75892-3   (eBook)
https://doi.org/10.1007/978-3-319-75892-3

Printed on acid-free paper

This Springer imprint is published by the registered company Springer International Publishing AG part of Springer Nature
The registered company address is: Gewerbestrasse 11, 6330 Cham, Switzerland

This small work is dedicated with eternal gratitude to the Lord our God, to his Son Jesus Christ, and to our blessed Mother the Holy Virgin Mary for allowing me to serve our ill and sick brothers and sisters to the full extent of my limited abilities.

To my wife, my critic and encouraging partner in this endeavor.

To our highly professional outstanding operating room nurses.

To our surgical Physician Assistants (PA) and Nurse Practitioners for their invaluable professional help and dedication in caring for our patients.

About the Author

J. Ernesto Molina is a native of Guatemala. He graduated from Medical School at the Universidad de San Carlos de Borromeo in Guatemala Cumma Sum Laude, receiving the Gold Medal "Flores Award" for his graduation thesis. He was Resident and Instructor of Surgery at University Hospital in Guatemala and recipient of the German scholarship from the Deutscher Akademisher Austaushdienst at the University of Düsseldorf. He completed his Surgery Residency in General and Cardiothoracic Surgery along with training in Cardiac Pathology and Physiology at the University of Minnesota. He received his Ph.D. in Surgery from the University of Minnesota. He is currently Full Professor of Surgery and Emeritus Professor of Cardiothoracic Surgery at the University of Minnesota in Minneapolis, USA.

Contents

Part I
General Practical Techniques

Chapter 1
Closure of Skin Incisions

Closure of the surgical incision after the operation has been completed is always important because is the first impression that the patient receives when he/she wakes up from anesthesia. For many years the use of the "steri-strips" was widely applied, hoping that by the time the strips start to fall off or are removed, the incision may be completely healed. However the strips leave a gooey sticky adhesive on the skin which is difficult to clean. An alternative was introduced with the use of metal staples which not only are painful to remove but also require special instrument to accomplish the task. Today fortunately the manner in which the skin incision is closed has changed significantly for the benefit of the patient. New methods have evolved aiming for more esthetic results leaving less visible scar along with a decrease of the risk of infection by using minimal dressing that does not require replacement and in addition, no pain is associated with the incision care. Therefore towards those goals most recently the implementation of the subcuticular suture is now in general application. After the incision is closed the following step is to apply what is called a liquid bandage which dries upon contact with the room air. This compound is applied with the pen-like applicator leaving a thin layer that does not require any dressing over it. Some trade names of such compounds are Dermabond, Skin Shield, Surgiseal, and others. The suture material used for the subcuticular suture consists of fine absorbable material like Vicryl, Dexon, Maxon, and others. However the technique to place a subcuticular suture has to follow certain principles that often are not observed. We have to explain that the idea is to have the incision nicely closed without leaving any material outside for later removal. To accomplish this requirement, the person doing the sawing begins the stich at the corner of the incision in the subcuticular level but tying it at that level. From there, the suture is run toward the other of the incision and upon reaching it the suture is again tied at that level. Even though the operator claims that the knot is placed in a deeper plane, this is never totally achieved.

© Springer International Publishing AG, part of Springer Nature 2018
J. E. Molina, *Cardiothoracic Surgical Procedures and Techniques*,
https://doi.org/10.1007/978-3-319-75892-3_1

The inconvenience of doing so is that as the suture material dissolves (absorbed) in the body, the knots don't dissolve at the same rate as the rest of the suture, and the bulky material migrates to the surface producing serous exudate with exposure of the knot which needs to be removed. Sometimes this is followed by limited partial dehiscence of the incision. This complication occurs because knots should not be present at the subcuticular level. Once the knots migrate to the surface, it causes staining of the patient's clothes which urges the patient to return for consultation to the clinic, implying, besides inconvenience, new expense of medical costs associated with the visit. This occurrence defeats the main purpose of using this closure method of not having exteriorized sutures to be removed in the postoperative follow-up.

The technique that avoids these minor problems is shown in the adjoined illustrations (Figs. 1.1, 1.2, and 1.3).

After the subcutaneous plane has been closed, the next step is to implement the superficial skin suture which is not subcuticular nor sub-dermic. The suture goes **intradermic** which constitutes the more firm fibrous layer of the skin below the epidermis. The suture is started by anchoring the stich deeper in the subcutaneous layer plane. The stich is tied there, and therefore the knot is deep. From there the suture is brought up to the dermic layer in the corner and it is now run parallel within the dermic layer to the end of the incision. The suture is not tied at that corner; instead the suture is advanced in the subcutaneous tissue exiting at least 1 in. away from the end corner. At that point, the suture is tied to itself as shown in the illustration (Fig. 1.3). As the knot is snugged we have three strands: the loop and the main suture exiting from the skin. Make sure to leave sufficient length to have this suture snipped later (usually 5–6 days) exerting gentle traction before cutting it at the skin level. At that point the healing is complete. Now a thin layer of Dermabond is applied over the incision. If the surgical incision is short, there is no need for dressings over it. The Dermabond film takes about 2 weeks to fall off by itself. There is no need to remove it.

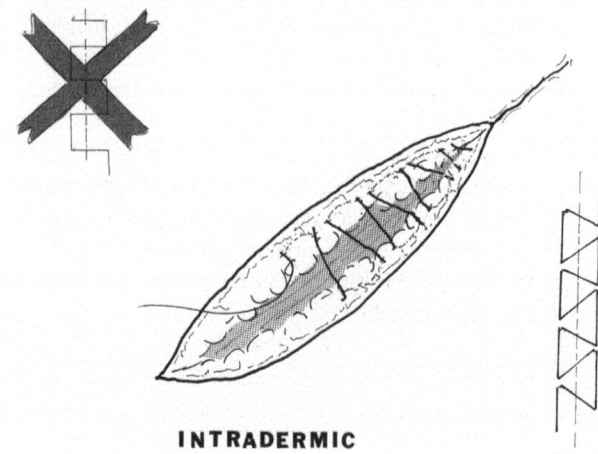

Fig. 1.1 Intradermic suture shown with the recommended pattern depicted on the right

INTRADERMIC

Fig. 1.2 The end of the suture brought out about 1 in. from the end of the incision. A manual tie is made keeping tension on the suture

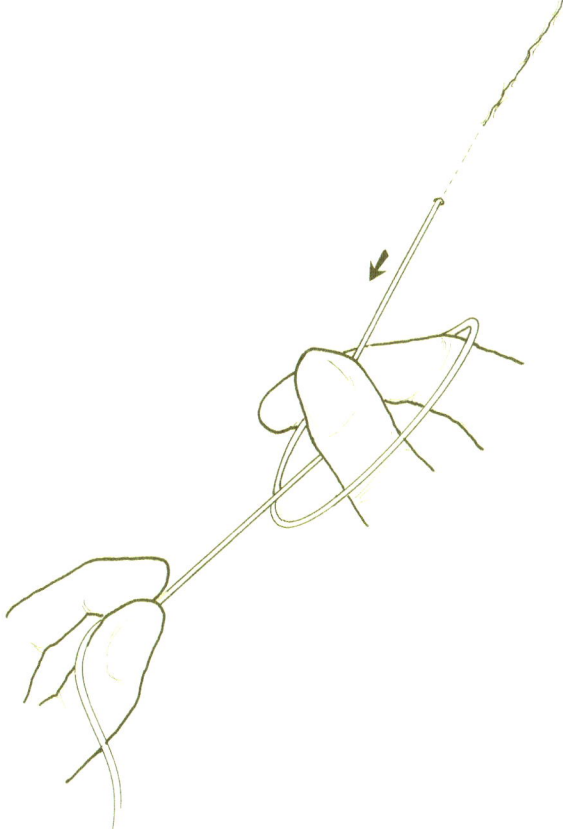

The second very important point is the manner in which the intradermic suture is handled. As the parallel suture runs it should not cross to the opposite side at a right angle because it would leave a small space which may evert when the suture is pulled snug. Instead when going to the other side the bite is placed back just next to the previous suture site. This is shown in the first illustration (Fig. 1.1).

When the incision is long and two surgeons are sawing from each corner, at the time they meet in the center, both sutures should exit the skin in the lower or in the upper side of the main incision away from the suture line and each suture is handled in the same manner as explain above.

This type of skin closure is applied to all surgical incisions including thoracotomies, sternotomies, and neck and abdominal incisions.

Fig. 1.3 The suture is tied
to itself bringing the knot
to the skin level shown on
the left and the suture is
cut leaving sufficient
length for future removal.
Dermabond is spread over
the incision that seals it

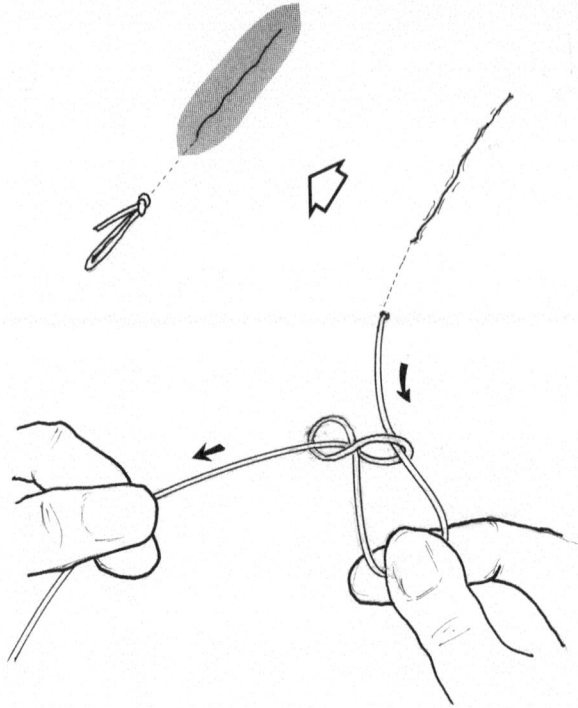

Chapter 2
Securing Cannula and Tube Connections

Placement of drains is a common practice in all types of surgeries. The drains usually have to stay in the patient for various periods of time. Other devices like cannulas are inserted for specific function during the conduct of an operation and removed as the operative procedure concludes. This situation is observed while implementing circulatory bypass procedures diverting the normal circulation in another direction to allow the intended corrective operation to be undertaken. In the area of thoracic surgery a chest tube drain is implanted in the chest cavity at the end of the operation to allow re-expansion of the lung that has been kept partially collapsed. One or more tubes can be used for that purpose. Those are brought out of the chest cavity through an intercostal space and are secured to the skin to prevent migration or dislodgement.

The usual method is to place a stitch at the skin opening constricting the skin around the tube to obliterate any possible air leak. Then, with the long tails of the suture, the chest tube is tied around snug enough to prevent its displacement. A simple knot with few more throws may be sufficient. However if the first tie is not tight enough, no matter how many more throws are placed afterwards, the tube will not be secured enough and may slide out later on. Therefore the emphasis here is on placing the first tie correctly.

Using a self-locking knot is the best faultless way to solve this problem and always be sure that the tube is perfectly secure. The steps to apply this tying maneuver are shown in the adjunct illustrations. By using the tails of the skin stitch already tied, the suture is taken twice around the tube as shown in the illustrations (Figs. 2.1, 2.2, 2.3, 2.4, 2.5, and 2.6). As the ends are pulled the tube is snuggly held fast and without keeping the free ends under tension the suture stays fast. As an extra measure one or two more throws can be added. The tube is now secured.

Now the tube must be connected to the suction draining unit which should be already functioning. The end of the chest tube has to be tailored at its distal end which is expanded, to receive the rigid connector of the collecting chamber tube. This is usually a tapered graded plastic piece. Once the chest tube is firmly hooked the connection is reinforced by placing a tie or the hospital may have the called

© Springer International Publishing AG, part of Springer Nature 2018
J. E. Molina, *Cardiothoracic Surgical Procedures and Techniques*,
https://doi.org/10.1007/978-3-319-75892-3_2

Fig. 2.1 The string is passed around the connecting tube to be secured

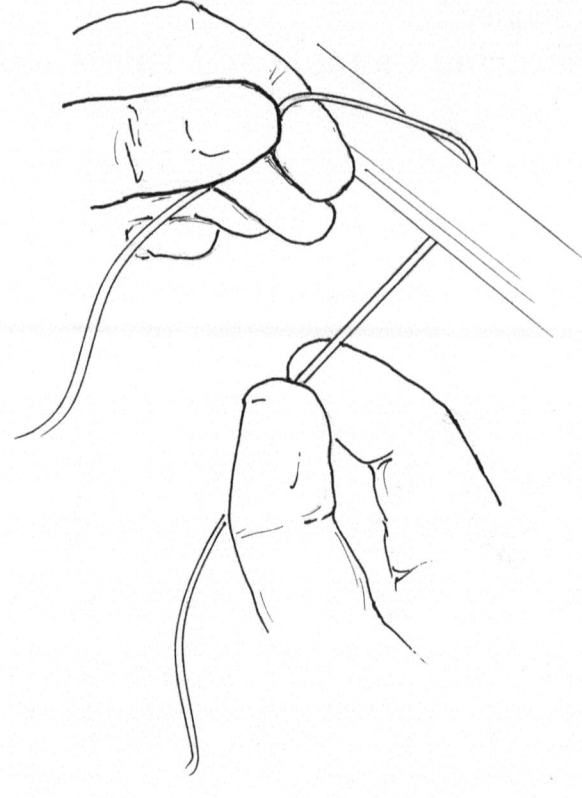

Fig. 2.2 The string is passed around a second time

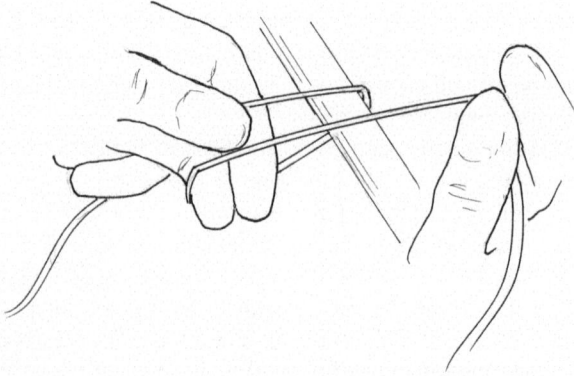

Fig. 2.3 The two loops of the suture are kept around the two left fingers and the tube

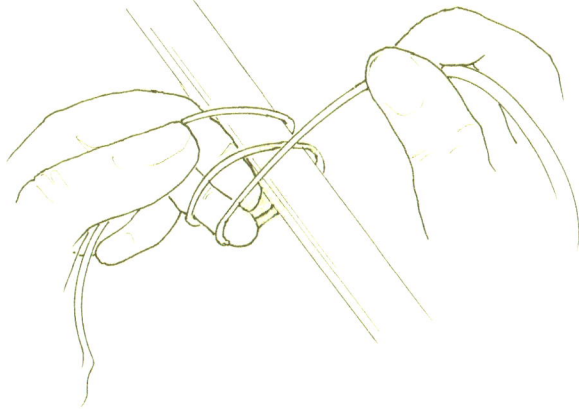

Fig. 2.4 Now the string is passed inside the two loops as shown and the fingers let the suture go

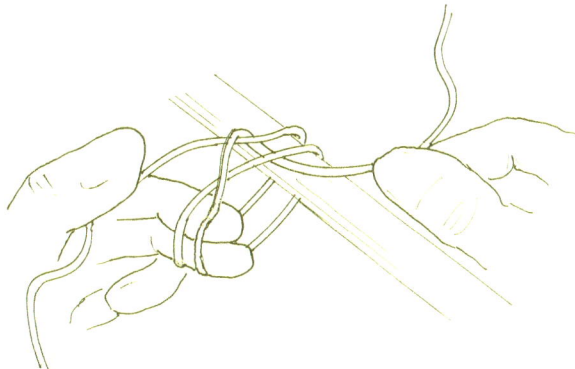

Fig. 2.5 Shows the detail on how the tying string is positioned inside the two loops of suture material

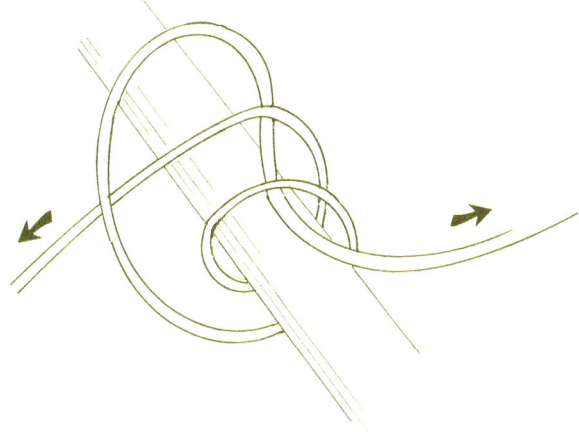

Fig. 2.6 The two ends of
the suture are pulled tight.
The knot stays secure and
will never loosen. One or
two additional throws may
be added for safety

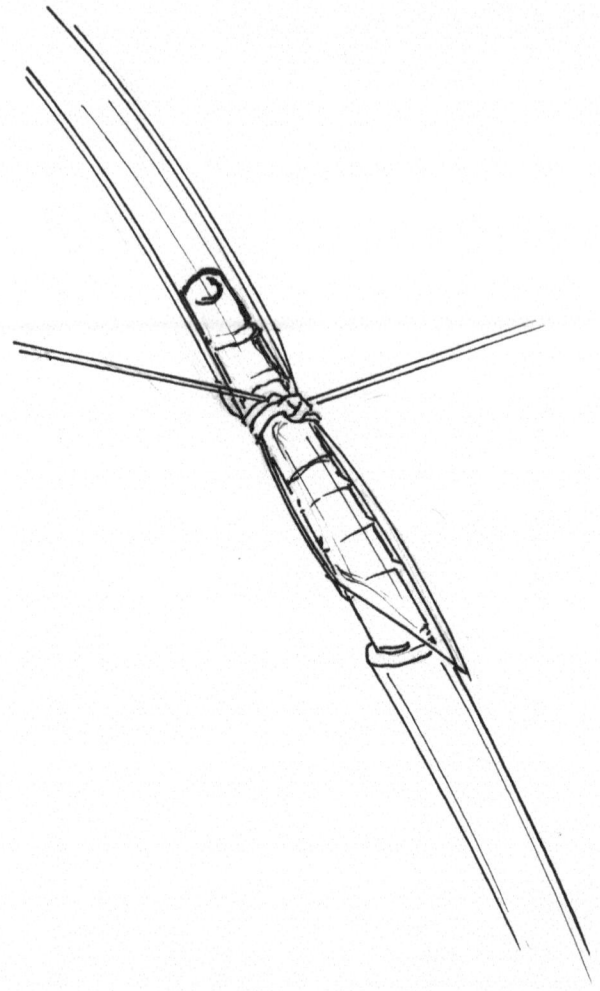

Tie Gun that uses plastic cable ties. Even using these plastic cables the tubes may
slip apart when the tension of the Tie Gun has not been set to the proper pulling
strength. Therefore the application of a self-locking knot with a heavy suture material gauge 0 or thicker even size 5 is preferable and never fails.

Occasionally when the patient is on the regular hospital ward and the chest tube
connection falls apart the ones who are called are the physician assistant (PA) or
Resident physician. All they have to do is to request or carry a package of heavy
suture material, Ethibond, Tevdek, or equivalent, and proceed to reconnect the tubes
and place a self-locking knot on the connection. Besides solving that problem, they
must request a chest X-ray study to see if the lung has collapsed.

Intraoperatively conducting cardiac operations and in particular open cardiac procedures with extracorporeal circulation the cannulas implanted to implement the bypass circuit need to be secured in place. These are aortic, atrial, left ventricular vents and cannulas to administer cardioplegic solutions. All of them are accompanied by a tourniquet that constricts the tissues around the insertion site to seal any leaks. The tourniquet is tied secured to each cannula with a reliable tie for the entire course of the operation. The best way to secure the cannula and the tourniquet is to use this same self-locking knot for which a suture 2-0 provides the adequate strength to secure both items without collapsing the cannula. One operator holds the cannula and tourniquet together while the other operator places the tie.

One last fact is that the knot cannot be loosened once placed. The circumference portion of the string tie must be cut to release the structures.

Chapter 3
Drainage of Pleural Effusions

Collection of fluid in the pleural cavity may occur from a wide variety of conditions. If no history of trauma exists or history of previous surgical interventions then the cause must be investigated. Among the possibilities we have to consider are pulmonary infections like pneumonia and malignancy of lymphatic origin. Most commonly however pleural effusions are associated with postoperative occurrences following cardiac interventions or pulmonary operations. Other causes which may pass undetected are previous intravenous implants of central catheters placed for therapeutic long-term infusion of antibiotics, for nutritional purposes when normal oral alimentation cannot be accomplished. Implant of dialysis catheters and also implant of pacemaker or defibrillator leads. During the implant of these devices particularly the antiarrhythmic leads may perforate the endocardium of the cardiac muscle with or without perforating the epicardium. Also occasionally a central catheter has gone the wrong path and has entered the mediastinal pleura. Other more common causes are a late complication following a cardiac surgical procedure which has apparently healed well but a few days or weeks later the patient is found with a pleural effusion in his/her follow-up chest radiographic study. This is not unusually seen in patients who have undergone cardiac valve replacement and are kept on chronic anticoagulation regimen. It also may occur when the chest tubes implanted at the time of surgery remain in the patient for several days but sometimes are removed too soon and the fluid continues to accumulate days later after the patient has been discharged from the hospital.

Another type of pleural effusion constitutes the presence of chylothorax. The continuous accumulation of lymph occurs when small lymphatic channels rupture or are injured during the operation but is not detected until few days later. The treatment of this condition is being addressed in the next chapter on the management of chest tubes and also in the chapter dedicated to the treatment of chylothorax.

It is, therefore, important to know the type of effusion to be treated.

With a simple tap with a needle and syringe, under local anesthesia the quality of the effusion is diagnosed. This is the first step and the most important to decide the proper treatment. Clear and tinged fluid effusion can be treated by simple drainage

© Springer International Publishing AG, part of Springer Nature 2018
J. E. Molina, *Cardiothoracic Surgical Procedures and Techniques*,
https://doi.org/10.1007/978-3-319-75892-3_3

with needle or small catheter. However if blood clots are present or fibrinous or purulent materials are present, only diagnostic puncture is justified. The patient most likely will need a thoracotomy to evacuate the pleural cavity and allow re-expansion of the lung.

The clear or amber-colored fluid is the most common finding. Also the blood-tinged fluid is commonly found in the patients who have had cardiac or thoracic surgery. This type of effusion is easily treated following the recommendation explained here.

Once the pleural effusion is diagnosed and verified by X-ray study, the fluid should be removed promptly to allow full re-expansion of the partially collapsed lung because gradually the pleura outlining the effusion begins to fibrose and impairs the lung re-expansion. This should not be allowed because if the lung remains trapped inside the chest cavity unable to expand, the patient will need to have a major operation named decortication. This is a difficult major undertaking and with some risks that will lay the patient in the hospital for several days. Therefore any pleural effusion, as soon as is diagnosed, needs to be treated immediately by draining it. Puncturing the pleura initially to make the diagnosis is very important to establish the etiology of the effusion. If the patient is still hospitalized, one option is to have the radiologist with the help of ultrasound to drain the fluid by inserting—what is called—a "pigtail catheter." This small line can be connected to a draining collecting chamber and left in place for 1–2 days until the drainage stops and then it is removed.

However, if the patient is being seen in an ambulatory or outpatient clinic, a simple and safe method is here illustrated that accomplishes the task avoiding the risk of puncturing the lung in the process (Fig. 3.1).

Under local anesthesia a long enough needle gauge 20 is fitted with an "IV extension tubing" which at the other end is connected to a large syringe provided with a three-way stopcock and another tubing leading to the collecting container. This method gives the needle free movement as the lung expands and while the diaphragm also moves superiorly. There is no pressure on the needle; therefore no puncture of the lung can occur. As the amount of fluid diminishes the needle can be removed gradually out (Fig. 4.1). Consequently trying to drain a pleural effusion with a syringe attached directly to the needle and the three-way stopcock is not recommended because if the needle injures the lung a more serious problem is created, namely the creation of pneumothorax. As stated, this additional injury could happen due to the repetitive maneuvers of manipulating the three-way stopcock aspirating and ejecting the fluid. The operator continuously transmits movements to the syringe while manipulating the three-way stopcock.

When draining a pleural effusion, the patient needs to be in a sitting position on the examining table and his/her arms and upper body rested over a Mayo stand with a pillow in order to have him/her rested and as comfortable as possible. The person assisting the operator, namely the nurse, must be making sure that the fluid is properly collected and all is handled properly under sterile conditions.

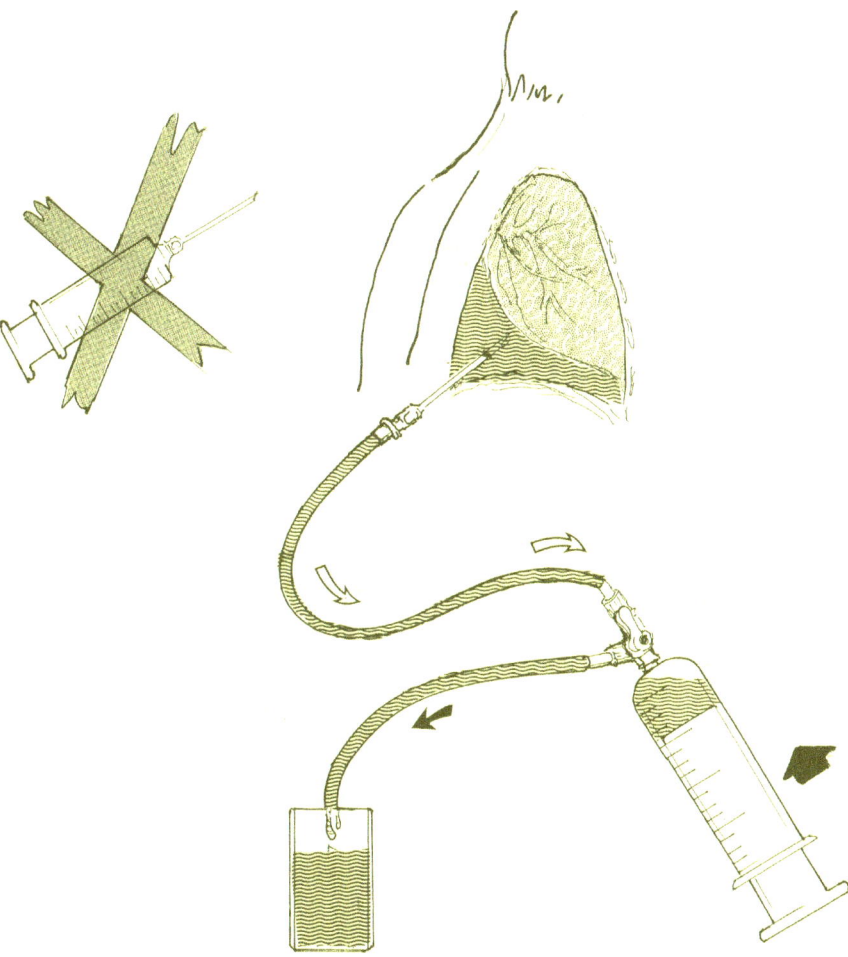

Fig. 3.1 The puncturing needle is connected to a short piece of extension IV tubing. Not directly to the syringe. The tubing is connected to a three-way stopcock and the syringe that can freely aspirate and eject the fluid to a container without transmitting the movements to the needle

Chapter 4
Insertion and Removal of Chest Tubes

As explained in the previous chapter, chest tube insertion is needed to treat large pleural effusions or acute purulent type which constitutes a pleural empyema. Sometimes an original effusion had been already drained but it had recurred. These cannot be treated with needle drainage or with small catheter implant. Usually complete drainage of such effusions takes several days and a formal chest tube insertion is required. Malignant effusions or chylothorax constitutes another indication for chest tube drainage.

Depending on the viscosity of the fluid the proper caliber of the tube is selected taking into consideration that the tube will have to stay in place for several days. If the radiological images show the presence of blood clots, the patient will need a formal thoracotomy to evacuate what is called a clotted hemothorax.

Chest tube insertion can be done by an interventional radiologist but this depends on the services available in the hospital. The radiologist guided by ultrasound or CT scan can puncture the site and using gradual dilators can adjust to the chest tube size to be inserted. However, often enough, particularly in postoperative situations, the patient is usually treated at the bedside by either the surgeon himself/herself or a resident physician, a fellow, or a physician assistant. Recommendations are given here to achieve a safe intervention, specifically aimed to avoid or prevent as much patient discomfort as possible. The procedure is done under local anesthesia with lidocaine hydrochloride (xylocaine) or similar anesthetic compound and the operator must verify whether the patient has allergies to these drugs to prevent any serious undesired reaction. The administration of a sedative is also recommended that would help to reduce the patient's anxiety.

© Springer International Publishing AG, part of Springer Nature 2018   17
J. E. Molina, *Cardiothoracic Surgical Procedures and Techniques*,
https://doi.org/10.1007/978-3-319-75892-3_4

Preparation

The operator must have an assistant, usually the nurse taking care of the patient. All the proper equipment should be in the room by the bedside to avoid trips back and forth, in and out of the room for items that were missing. The container to collect the drained fluid must be already connected to the suction line and functioning. The sterile tray with the instruments and materials needed should be placed on a Mayo stand or equivalent, at the bedside but not open at this point. The tray should contain the following items:

Sterile towels	5
Needle driver	1
Surgical sutures Ethibond size 2-0 on a swaged taper-point needle	2
Heavy tubing clamp	1
Rankin hemostatic forceps	2
Hypodermic syringe 20 cc size, and needles 25, 20, 21	1
Gauze pads 4 × 4 and 2 × 2	4
Scalpel and blades 10 and 15 (or 11)	1
Scissors	1
Sterile glass shot (to receive the antiseptic solution)	1

Available in the room but not included in the sterile tray: xylocaine solution vial of 100 mL; sterile surgical glove sizes 7, 71/2, and 8; antiseptic solution (Betadine, Hibiclens, or similar); antibiotic or iodine ointment that will be applied to the skin incision at the entry site of the tube; Ethibond free ties size 0; dressing and adhesive tape; chest tubes of the selected size: 24–28. Usually there is no need to insert tubes of larger diameter.

Chest Tube Implant

With the patient lying in a comfortable position, exposing the side of the chest where the tube will be implanted, the selected point is determined. After the surgical field is aseptically treated, local anesthetic is injected subcutaneously for a length of about 2 in. along the intercostal space selected. From that point using a longer hypo-dermic needle a track of approximately 4 to 5 cm (2 1/2 to 3 in.) long is also infil-trated further along the same space. The intercostal muscle and the pleura are also infiltrated. The minimal amount of anesthetic needed is 20 mL. Do not plan on inserting the tube riding over the next upper rib. This is wrong and causes severe pain afterwards because the tube is kinked and is continuously being pinched between the ribs with the respiratory movements. The tube should enter the chest cavity in the same space where the initial incision was made (Figs. 4.1, 4.2, and 4.3). Once the tunnel is created with the Rankin forceps, the pleural cavity is entered, and

Fig. 4.1 A small incision
is made in the skin, at the
site where the chest tube is
to be inserted

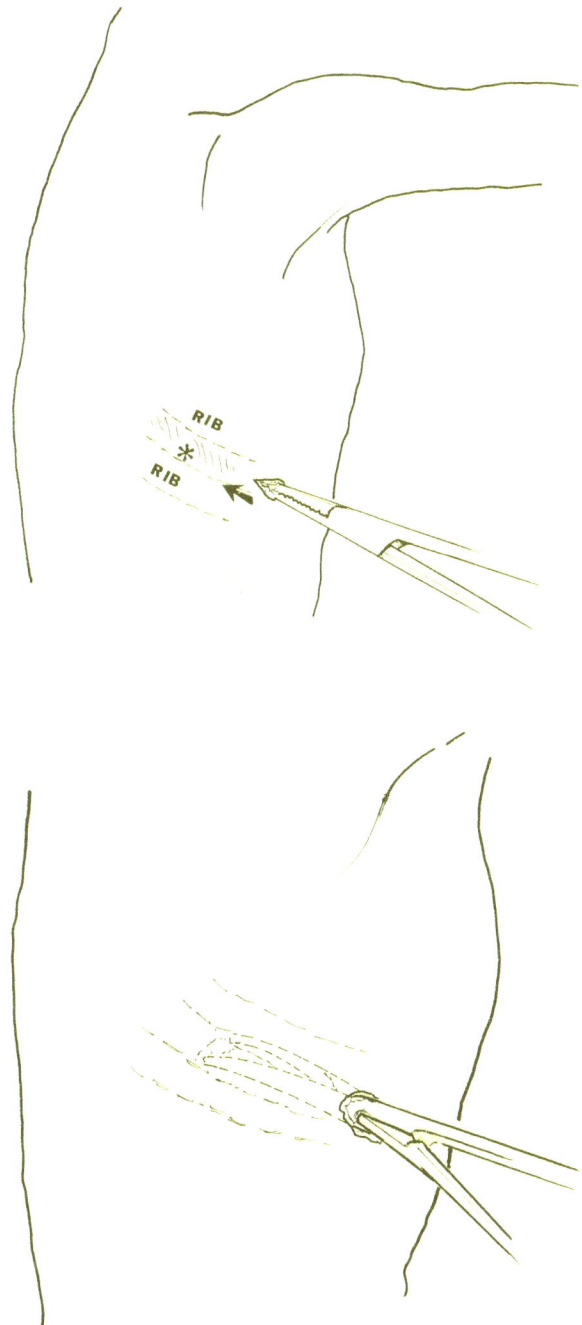

Fig. 4.2 With a hemostatic
forceps a tunnel is created
about 4 cm long to the
level where the chest tube
will enter the chest cavity

Fig. 4.3 Now the chosen
chest tube is guided held
with the forceps and
inserted in the chest cavity
at the end of the tunnel.
The tube must have a
clamp placed in the distal
portion to prevent any
splashing of fluid or blood
in the field

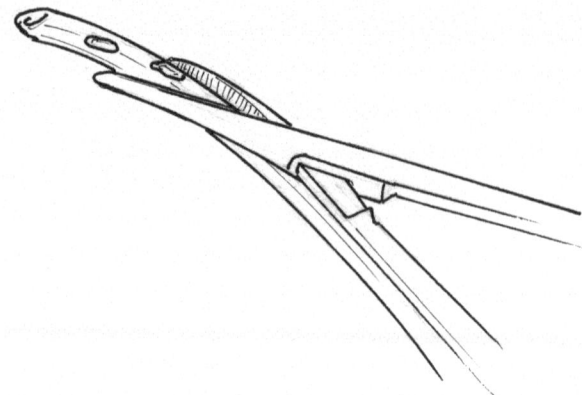

the opening is enlarged by spreading the forceps jaws. The chest tube is under sterile conditions handed over by the nurse. One of the heavy tubing clamps is applied to the distal end before insertion to prevent fluid splash in the field. Now the Rankin forceps holds the tip of the tube which is guided through the subcutaneous tunnel and driven into the pleural cavity. The forceps is removed while the tube is advanced into the chest. The operator makes sure that the tube is freely sliding in and out into the thoracic cavity. The tube is now secured to the skin by placing the skin stitch with Ethibond 2-0. The skin stitch should be wide and placed in such a manner that snugs the skin around the tube. With the same suture the tube is tied as well to secure it to the chest wall. The tube is now connected to the suction system and only now the clamp placed on the distal tube is released. Fluid and air will drain rapidly in the container. Antibiotic ointment and dressings are applied over the site of insertion. The patient is asked to take deep breaths and cough to help evacuate the fluid.

Removal of the Tube

Removal of the chest tube when no longer needed should follow a few precautions to prevent the development of pneumothorax. This is the most common complication during this maneuver, particularly when the task is delegated to personnel with limited experience handling this simple maneuver. What is commonly seen is having the operator ask the patient to exert some pressure by closing their mouth and pressing down while the tube is quickly removed. Some patient can comply with this request but for others it does not work because they are not able to do it at satisfaction. To avoid placing this responsibility on the patient, there is a safe simple maneuver to follow without the patient's participation. This is the method:

All the current chest draining systems consist of a chamber that regulates the vacuum or suction imposed to the draining unit that is called "negative pressure" implemented by a water seal system. Most of the time the system is set to 20 mm of suction which is maintained by the water seal level that bubbles continuously. The

Fig. 4.4 At the time of removal, the assistant (nurse) occludes digitally the vent orifices of the collecting container at the moment the tube is rapidly removed

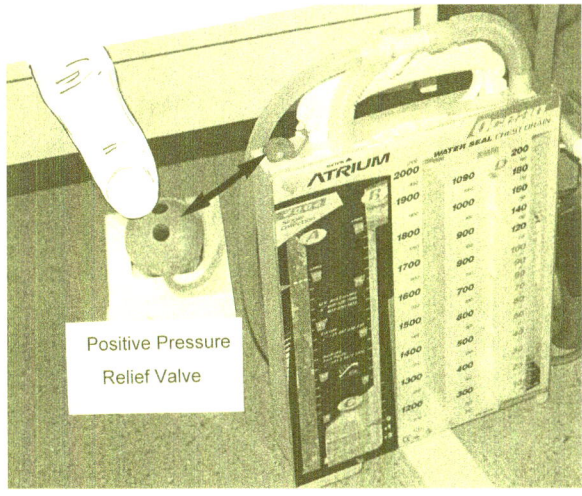

Positive Pressure
Relief Valve

chamber unit has one or two holes at the top which is the site that regulates the func-tion. To remove the chest tube from the patient, the operator needs the help of the nurse to implement the maneuver (Fig. 4.4). When the tube is ready to come out and the suture holding the tube to the chest wall has been released, the operator grabs the tube with one hand and with the other hand a dressing with sufficient amount of Betadine or antibiotic ointment is pressed over the orifice on the skin. At this moment without changing the wall suction, which should stay on, the nurse is asked to occlude with her finger the vent orifice of the chamber (Fig. 4.4). This maneuver places strong vacuum on the tube which is now simultaneously rapidly removed. The skin opening is occluded with the dressing containing the ointment. There is no problem implementing this maneuver and no blame can be placed on the operator, being this a resident or physician assistant giving that mission.

In the cases when the chest tube drainage unit does not use the water seal equip-ment like the Thopaz (Medela Inc.), which operates with an electrical mechanism, the vacuum can be increased while removing the chest.

Part II
Thoracic Surgical Procedures and Techniques

Chapter 5
Thoracotomy

Although the word thoracotomy implies any type of operation surgically entering the chest cavity, in this section only the standard incision made to expose the thoracic internal organs without any modifications like extending the incisions involving division of the sternum or entering the abdomen is addressed. Depending on the magnitude of the planned intervention, the length of the incision varies according to the amount of exposition needed to allow manual manipulations, or the introduction of mechanical devices like staplers necessary to accomplish the proposed task.

The patient is positioned in lateral decubitus with the side of the chest to be intervened up. The thoracic incision is made following the direction of the ribs. Usually the most frequent levels are over the fourth, fifth, or sixth ribs. The most common target organs are the lungs, esophagus, thoracic aorta, and mediastinum. After the skin and the subcutaneous tissues, the muscular layers must be retracted or divided to expose the rib cage. At that time the decision must be made on how to proceed to enter the chest cavity. Potentially two techniques could be implemented.

One option is by entering the chest through the intercostal space which in general is not the best nor the recommended technique. If this is decided the intercostal muscles along with the pleura are incised just following the superior border of the rib. The disadvantages of this approach are several: First of all this slice offers very limited area to obtain adequate exposure, inadequate for digital and even less for manual manipulation. Placement of a mechanical retractor often leads to rib fracture while trying to enlarge the area of work. Along with that inconvenience also the incision is often extended in both directions tearing more muscle. At the end of the operation the closure on the incision is achieved by placing strong sutures **around** the ribs to bring them together, but the sutures going around the inferior rib invariably constrict the intercostal bundle nerve and vessels. To accomplish airtight closure the ribs are pulled until they touch each other. In addition the amount of soft muscular tissues does not present an identifiable adequate strong edge to seal off the incision. All those maneuvers are translated to a very painful postoperative evolution. Therefore for the reasons explained above, the plain intercostal incision cannot be recommended as ideal.

© Springer International Publishing AG, part of Springer Nature 2018
J. E. Molina, *Cardiothoracic Surgical Procedures and Techniques*,
https://doi.org/10.1007/978-3-319-75892-3_5

A second more acceptable technique is described here that involves the removal of the rib that provides a more satisfactory open space without excessive spreading of the rib cage. At the time of closure it allows for a more esthetically acceptable and precise repair.

To achieve and conduct this thoracotomy technique the following steps need to be taken. As the rib cage is exposed, a subperiosteal resection of the selected rib is undertaken. An incision is made with the cautery in the center of the rib to the entire length from one end to the other. With a periosteal elevator the upper and the lower layers are stripped with a sweeping movement, the upper side going from the back to the front and the lower side from the front to the back. The periosteum is detached in the back as well until the rib is totally isolated. Now the rib is excised and removed from the field. The remaining layer is now formed by the periosteum and the pleura which are entered and the chest cavity is open. It is now easier to position a rib retractor to expose the desired area. The opening allows for the necessary exploration and manipulations, and evacuation of blood clot if a clotted hemothorax was being treated. The intercostal vessels and nerves of the upper and lower ribs are left intact. The practice of purposely removing the intercostal nerve does not seem to have any beneficial effect.

The only situations in which this more elaborate technique may not be fully applicable are in emergency cases that require immediate control of a rupture vessel or aneurysm, and also in cases of gunshot or stab wounds that are life threatening representing life-or-death situations. The surgeon must use his/her judgment to use the quickest approach to deal with the problem. Injuries to the great vessels fall also in this category. The technique of how to close this type of thoracotomy is addressed in the following chapter.

Chapter 6
Closure of the Thoracotomy

The descriptions given in this chapter are applicable to the preferred type of thoracotomy presented in the previous chapter.

Once the thoracic operation is completed and providing that at this point a chest tube has been positioned in the chest cavity and secured in place for the postoperative period of observation, then closure of the thoracotomy is undertaken. This technique demonstrates two valid points of advantage over the only intercostal incision.

The inferior rib should be stripped of the periosteum without damaging the intercostal neurovascular bundle. Using a drill, three holes are made in the center of the rib at a proper distance from each other. Through these holes heavy sutures will be placed to approximate it to the upper rib. Depending on the size of the patient, nonabsorbable suture material size 2–5 Ethibond, Tevdek, Mersilene, etc. are passed around flush to the superior border of the upper rib and now through the drilled holes in the lower rib. At this point the sutures are not tied (Fig. 6.1). The next step follows.

The soft tissues comprising the intercostal muscles, periosteum, and pleura left from the resected rib are sutured in a single layer in a running fashion as follows: Two separate continuous sutures are started one at each end of the incision encircling the stump of the resected rib. The sutures are advanced toward the center of the incision but are not tightened but only laced until they meet in the center. Most commonly absorbable material is selected like Vicryl, Catgut, and Dexon of size 0–1. At this stage a metal rib approximator embracing the upper and lower ribs is placed that gradually brings the ribs closer, but only to a distance equivalent to the space that was occupied by the resected rib. This amounts to about half inch or one-and-a-half centimeters. The ribs should never be pulled to the point of touching each other (Fig. 6.2).

Now the heavy sutures placed around the ribs are pulled snug and tied secure. The rib approximator is removed and the next layer of soft tissues is closed. The

© Springer International Publishing AG, part of Springer Nature 2018
J. E. Molina, *Cardiothoracic Surgical Procedures and Techniques*,
https://doi.org/10.1007/978-3-319-75892-3_6

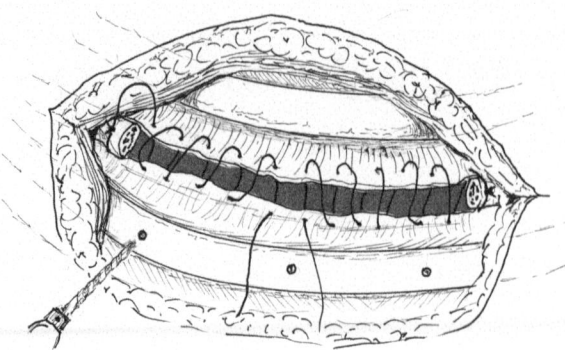

Fig. 6.1 Two steps are shown to close the thoracotomy: (**a**) Using a drill, three holes are made in the center of the inferior rib that is stripped off the periosteum preserving the integrity of the nerve and intercostal vessels. (**b**) Two running sutures are used to reapproximate the pleura, periosteum, and intercostal muscles of the resected rib starting on both ends of the incision without tightening them, but just loosely lacing them until they meet the center of the incision (see description in the text)

Fig. 6.2 Heavy sutures are placed around the upper rib and through the holes of the lower rib to approximate the ribs leaving a space between them equivalent to the distance that was occupied by the excised rib (about 2 cm)

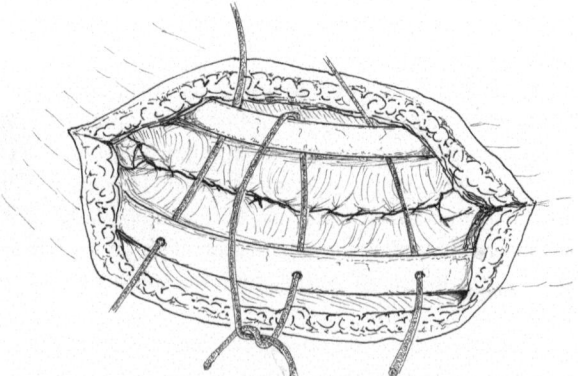

running sutures loosely placed in this layer are now gradually pulled snug, loop by loop, to seal the pleura with the periosteum and intercostal muscles of the excised rib. As they meet in the center of the incision, they are tied secure (Fig. 6.3). The remaining layers of the chest wall and skin are closed according to the preference of the surgeon. It is recommended however to close the skin as explained in Chap. 1 of this manual. With this technique there is no constriction of the intercostal nerve and therefore promoting less postoperative pain to the patient.

Fig. 6.3 Now the loose
sutures placed to close the
pleura and intercostal
muscles are pulled snug
loop by loop and tied in the
center of the incision

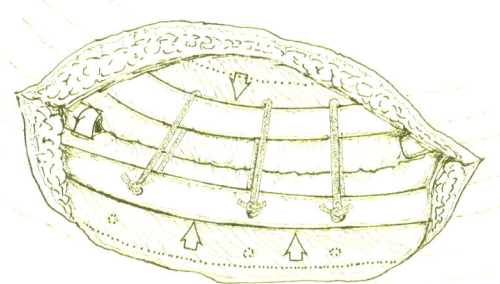

Chapter 7
Chronic Pleural Empyema

This constitutes a serious infection of the pleural cavity which most commonly occurs due to a previous acute empyema that was not properly treated. Whenever a pleural empyema is diagnosed, it should be promptly drained by insertion of a chest tube and simultaneous implementation of systemic antibiotic therapy. However if previously a pneumonectomy has been done, usually due to malignancy, the empty pleural cavity could become infected despite aggressive use of antibiotics topically and systemically that fails, and the treatment of temporary placement of chest tubes attempted also fails, the infection persists, and more drastic treatment will be needed. Techniques using large open chest tube drains anchored to the chest wall are uncomfortable to the patient and repeated irrigations of the pleural cavity are difficult to perform because of the tendency of the tube drainage to fall out.

Therefore a procedure to provide an effective permanent drainage and to facilitate daily irrigations without causing painful sessions of maintenance care is preferable. The creation of a permanent opening without tubes allows for easier care of the patient. The operation known as an Eloesser flap procedure named after its creator fulfills these conditions. The details for the proper application of this technique are mostly absent from the thoracic surgery books. Nevertheless the needed details are now here explained.

As a "sine qua non" condition, to create this type of drainage the mediastinum of the patient must be already rigid and chronically fibrosed to assure that the remaining opposite lung will not be compressed and that the respiratory function of the patient will not be further compromised.

Once the most dependent site of the pleural cavity is identified, an opening is created in the chest wall at that location by removing a segment of rib and constructing a flap with the soft tissues of the chest wall placing the skin layer inside the pleural cavity to prevent closure of the orifice by healing of the surrounding soft tissues.

© Springer International Publishing AG, part of Springer Nature 2018   31
J. E. Molina, *Cardiothoracic Surgical Procedures and Techniques*,
https://doi.org/10.1007/978-3-319-75892-3_7

Two types of flaps have been described in the literature:

1. An inferiorly based flap, anchoring the tip of the flap either to the diaphragmatic surface or around the inferior rib. The problem with this setup is that because of the thickness of the flap the irrigation of the cavity and the drainage is obstructed by the bulk of the flap and also securing the tip of the flap to the inside of the pleural cavity may be cumbersome and may fail.
2. On the other hand, a superiorly based thin soft-tissue flap is preferable to avoid the disadvantages of the inferiorly based type particularly if the flap is too thick. Therefore in the accompanied illustrations, the steps to implement this operation are shown (Figs. 7.1, 7.2, 7.3, 7.4, 7.5, 7.6, and 7.7).

A "U"-shaped incision is made over the level of the rib to be removed. The cut comprises all soft-tissue layers of the chest wall. This tongue-shaped portion is reflected upwards detaching it from the rib cage. However the flap so constructed must be thinned out by removing all the muscle tissue, leaving only the

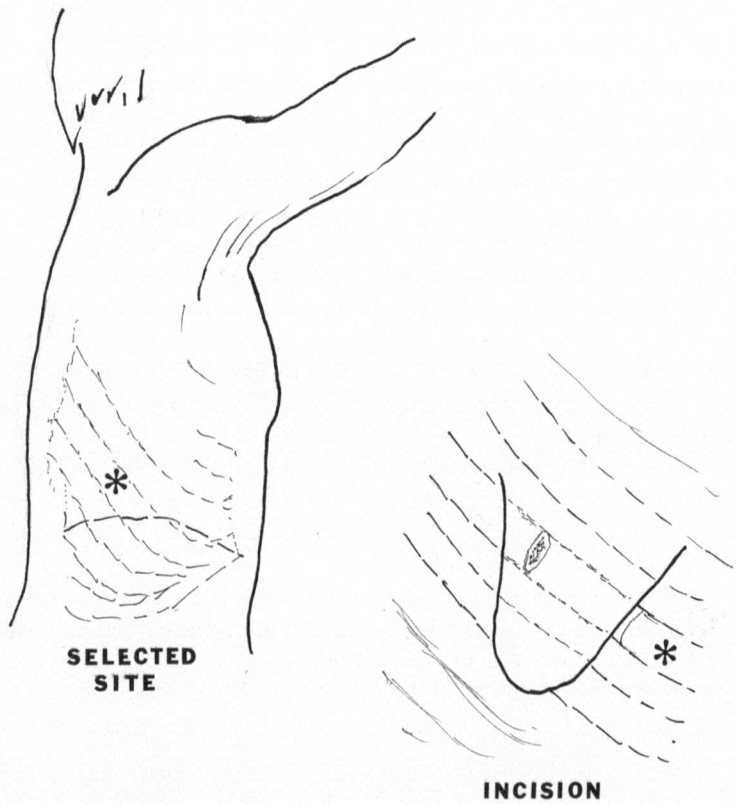

Fig. 7.1 A "U"-shaped incision is made at the most dependent level of the empyema over the selected rib to be removed

Fig. 7.2 The incision cuts through all chest wall layers but the muscle layer should be removed from the flap to make it thinner consisting only of skin and subcutaneous tissue

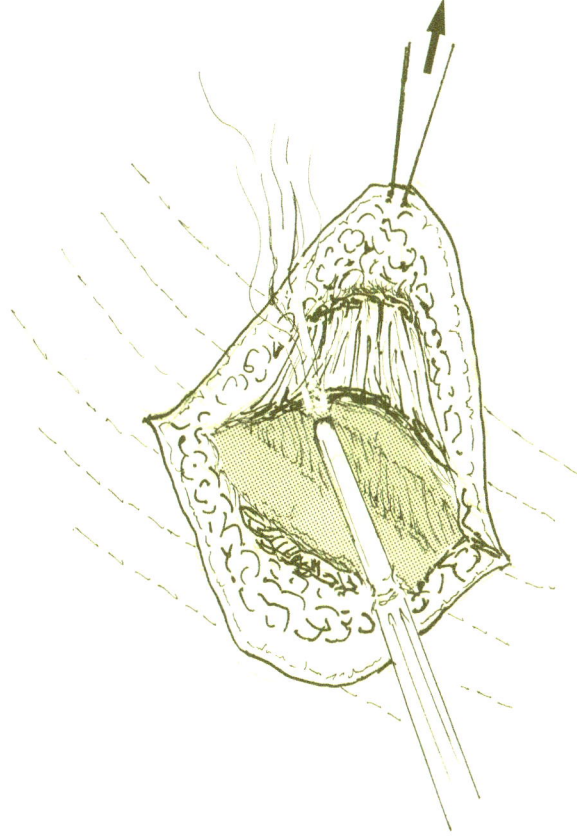

Fig. 7.3 The muscle is being removed and a subperiosteal resection of the rib is carried out

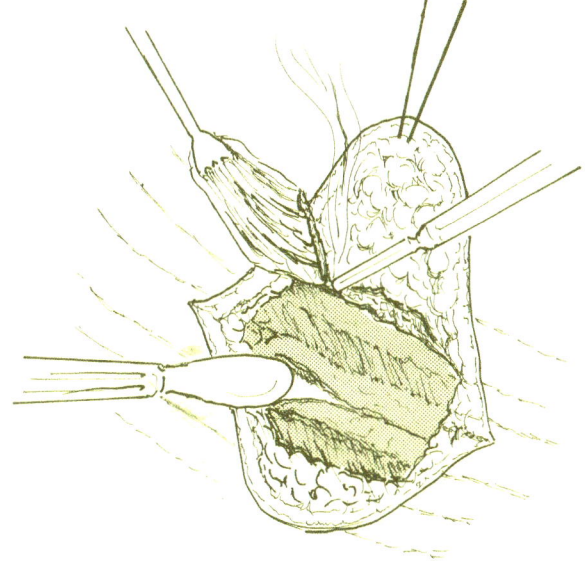

Fig. 7.4 The rib segment is resected and the flap is reflected up

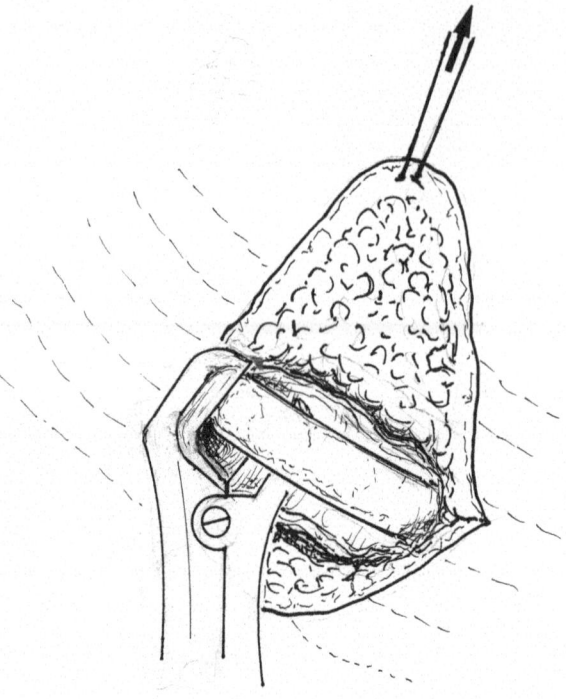

Fig. 7.5 The pleura has been entered, intercostal muscles are resected that create a round defect where the flap is inserted as shown

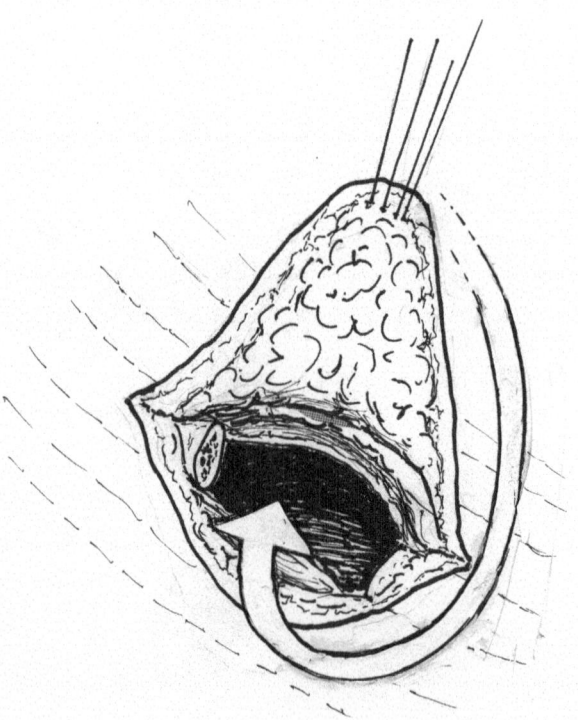

Fig. 7.6 Cross-section view of the chest wall showing the position of the Eloesser flap anchored to the inside of the chest cavity, and the large opening for drainage and irrigations

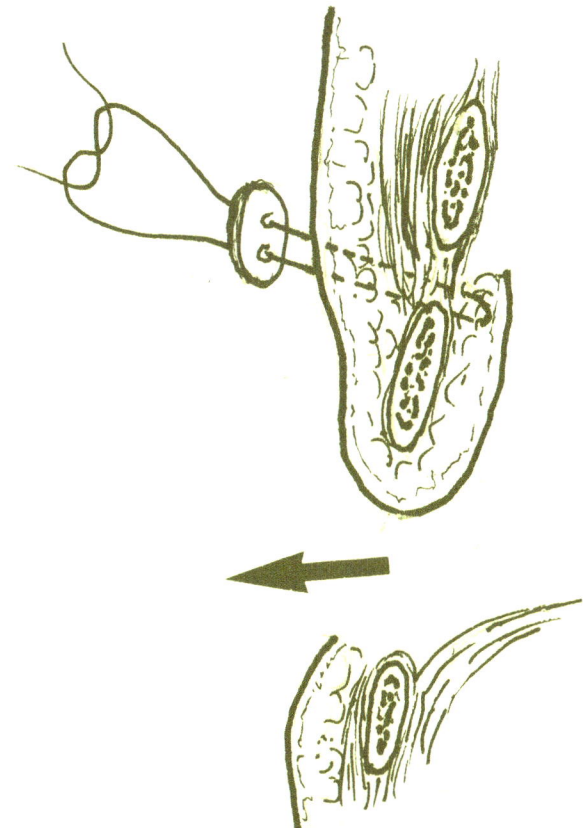

subcutaneous layer with the skin. Creating the flap in this manner will also facilitate its fixation to the chest wall inside the pleural cavity. Following the known surgical principles, the length of the flap should not be longer than the base in order to prevent ischemia.

Lifting this flap, the ribcage is exposed. The selected segment of rib is now resected. This is done by stripping the periosteum off the rib all the way around before dividing it and resecting it. After the rib is resected, the chest cavity is entered through the bed of the excised rib. The intercostal bundle must be ligated and divided at both ends and all the soft tissues are divided and resected creating a large opening into the chest cavity that the surgeon can explore digitally. The pleural cavity is irrigated thoroughly with antibiotic solution and all fibrinous material and debris are removed.

After the flap is thinned out, it is flipped inside the pleural cavity where it will be anchored. To fix the flap on the inside of the chest a monofilament suture (Prolene) size 0 or 2-0 swaged on to a taper-point large needle is passed from the outside through the chest wall just flush to the superior border of the next upper rib. The

Fig. 7.7 The final
completed aspect of the
operation

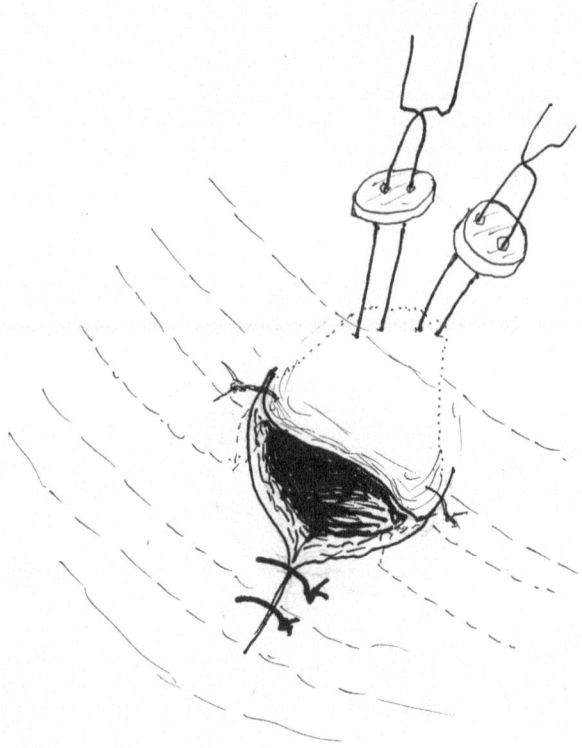

needle is retrieved from the inside of the chest and the tip of the flap is sutured with
one single passage making sure that the strong fibrous tissue is taken in it. Then the
same suture with the taper-point needle is passed from the inside of the chest cavity
to the outside over the upper rib. The two ends of the suture are threaded through a
retain button. A second suture is placed in the same manner next to the previous one.
Both sutures with retain buttons are tied. This will secure the flap to the chest wall
and the sutures are kept in place for at least 2 weeks. In undernourished patients the
sutures may have to stay longer. At the end of that period the stitches holding the
flap are removed. The edges of the lower end of the opening are approximated with
interrupted stitches of monofilament material. Dressings are applied but it is recommended that a dressing is applied utilizing what is called Montgomery straps that sit
somewhat away from the main incision where the gauze pads are held with twill ties
without removing the straps more than once a month. These dressing changes are
more practical on a daily basis as well as well tolerated. This avoids irritation of the
skin if regular tape is used every time the patient comes for dressing change.

Chapter 8
Pleurodesis

The obliteration of the pleural space is sometimes required as a therapeutic option to treat various conditions. One of them is the development of recurring spontaneous pneumothorax, which happens most frequently in chronic smokers, due to rupture of blebs on the surface of the lung. In cases of young nonsmokers it is probably due to congenital weakness of the visceral pleura. The first line of treatment is usually the insertion of a chest catheter to allow re-expansion of the lung. However if pneumothorax continues to recur two or more times the procedure called pleurodesis may be indicated, provided that no other pulmonary conditions requiring different specific therapy exist. In cases of malignancy already under treatment with recurrent pleural effusion, obliteration of the pleural cavity may be the only solution. Pleurodesis has also been implemented in the treatment of recurring chylothorax that has its origin following posterior mediastinal type of surgery like esophagus plastic intervention or resection. It may occur also as primary evolution of the lymphatic malignancy involving the mediastinal lymph nodes.

Currently to implement fusion of the pleural cavity does not require an open surgical procedure as was common practice in the past. Therefore the condition is effectively treated by injecting a chemical compound through a catheter or chest tube inserted in the pleural cavity by the techniques explained in the previous section of insertion of chest tubes. Several compounds have been used for this type of treatment, among them talc (injected as an emulsion) which is easy to obtain and prepare. Bleomycin and tetracycline can also be used. It appears that talc is the safest compound. Bleomycin has side effects and toxicity since it is a chemotherapeutic drug. Tetracycline may be difficult to obtain in a powder form to be used as a liquid solution.

Although in the past the previous infusion of a local anesthetic through the chest catheter was thought to minimize the pain caused by the injection of the therapeutic compound, the pain experienced by the patient is always severe and not effectively avoided. Therefore in my practice I have routinely requested to perform this treatment under what is called monitored anesthesia care (MAC) anesthesia to eliminate altogether the suffering of the patient. This type of anesthesia is not the same as

© Springer International Publishing AG, part of Springer Nature 2018 37
J. E. Molina, *Cardiothoracic Surgical Procedures and Techniques*,
https://doi.org/10.1007/978-3-319-75892-3_8

moderate sedation/analgesia (conscious sedation). "An essential component of MAC is the anesthesia assessment and management of a patient's actual or antici-pated physiological derangements or medical problems that may occur during this therapeutic modality. The provider of MAC must be prepared and qualified to con-vert to general anesthesia when necessary. By contrast, Moderate Sedation is not expected to induce depths of sedation that would impair the patient's own ability to maintain the integrity of his or her airway." The request to implement MAC anes-thesia must be strictly followed if we aim to avoid completely the discomfort always associated with this procedure as well as to secure the patient safety.

The sclerosing agent is injected slowly via the chest tube already in place. The tube is clamped while the drug is being injected and once the total amount is in the tube should remain clamped for several minutes (10–15 min) allowing the drug to spread in the pleural cavity. If feasible the patient position should be rotated or rolled, and maneuver aimed to have the medication evenly distributed to all areas of the chest cavity. The amount of fluid containing the drug varies from 20 to 50 mL.

After the session is completed the chest tube is unclamped and the fluid is allowed to drain in the chest tube container. On a daily basis the amount of drainage is measured until no more significant amount is obtained.

The draining fluid may stop altogether after one session, but if the amount of fluid only decreases but continues to drain a second injection may be required and the same sequence is followed. As no more drainage is measured, the chest tube is removed following the standard technique.

Chapter 9
Repair of Isolated Sternal Fracture

Isolated sternal fracture is a condition that occurs due to direct trauma to the front of the chest caused by falls, work-related injuries, or car accidents but without any damage to the internal organs. Severe trauma to the sternum most of the time is associated with injury of the inner organs and therefore care of these patients is directed to the most important and urgent life-threatening conditions like rupture of the aorta, lung injury, rupture of cardiac chambers, esophagus, and others. However most commonly the impact to the chest without any detectable damage of the internal organs happens when the anterior chest hits the steering wheel of the vehicle. In such cases, even though the radiographic evaluation reveals the fracture, this finding alone is not a condition that requires emergency repair and the patient is usually sent home with symptomatic treatment. Nevertheless repair of the fracture should be undertaken soon. If the patient is left to heal spontaneously he/she suffers physical deformity and chronic pain and adopts a slouch posture; it shows a bulge at the site of the fracture, and the patient has a restricted neck extension. When the sternum fractures, there is a downward migration of the superior portion of the bone that overlaps behind the lower half. The type of repair that is depicted in this section is recommended when no internal organ injury has occurred.

A simple chest X-ray study (Figs. 9.1 and 9.2) shows the radiologic and anatomical aspects of the fractured sternum with the overlap of the two portions.

To repair the fracture, the patient is positioned in supine position.

The proper anterior skin incision to expose the site of the fracture is equal for men and women (Figs. 9.3 and 9.4).

Dissection of the fragments is conducted using the cautery until the two segments are separated (Fig. 9.5).

Protecting the mediastinum with a flexible metal ribbon retractor (Fig. 9.6), using a drill, two holes are made in the upper and lower fragments of the sternum at an appropriate distance from the fracture gap to assure solid strength for placement of wire sutures that will bring the two halves together.

© Springer International Publishing AG, part of Springer Nature 2018
J. E. Molina, *Cardiothoracic Surgical Procedures and Techniques*,
https://doi.org/10.1007/978-3-319-75892-3_9

Fig. 9.1 Classical
radiological image of a
fractured sternum with the
two overlapping fragments.
The upper fragment under
the lower portion

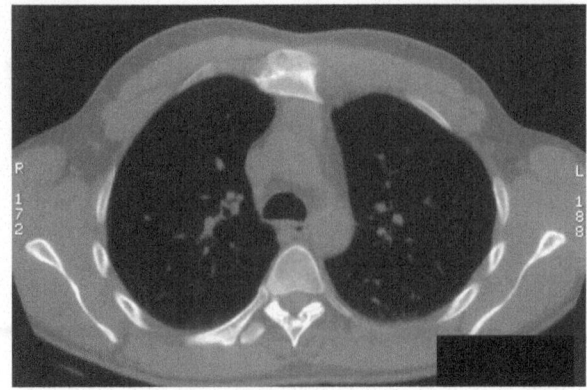

Fig. 9.2 Classical
radiological image of a
fractured sternum with the
two overlapping fragments.
The upper fragment under
the lower portion

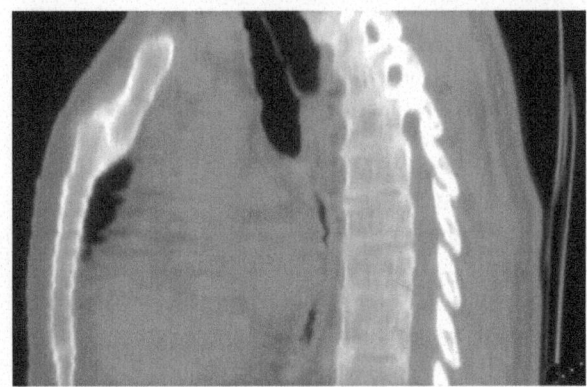

Fig. 9.3 The anterior
bilateral incision to
approach the fracture site

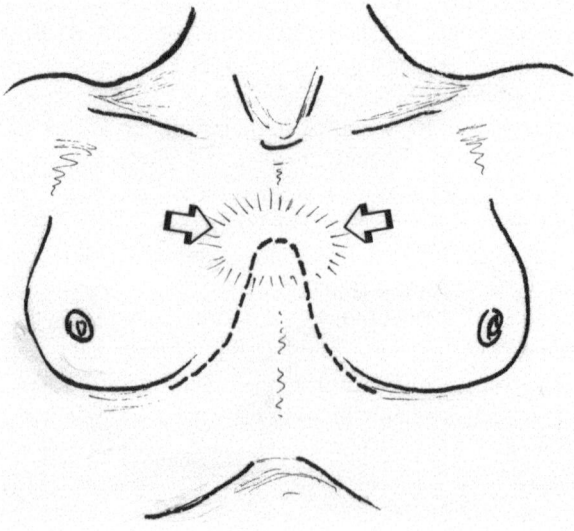

Fig. 9.4 The actual position of the fragments under the visible external bulge

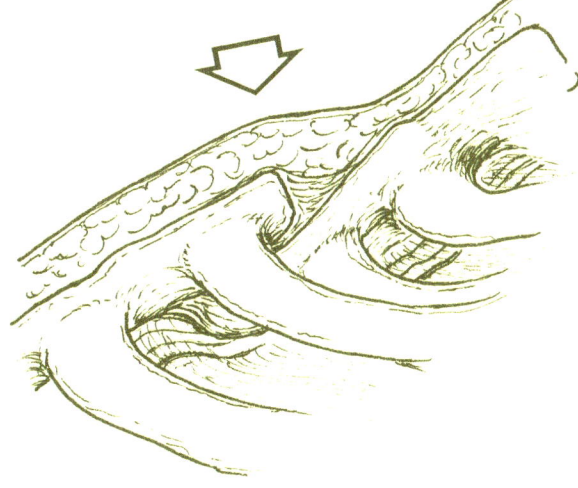

Fig. 9.5 The dissection and separation of the two sternal fragments using the cautery

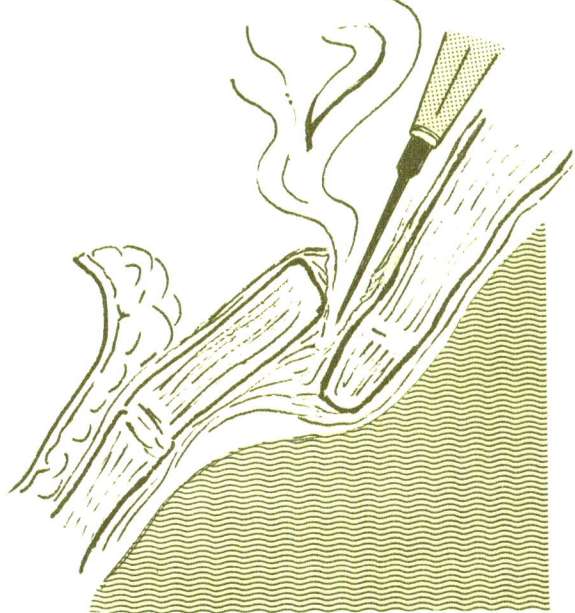

Depending on the situation, the internal thoracic vessel artery and vein need to be ligated.

When the two fragments are mobilized, help from the anesthesiologist is kindly requested. The operating table is positioned in a hyperextension mode to facilitate alignment of the fragments aimed to achieve strong proper anchoring end to end of both fragments. There is always a need to use large bone graspers (Fig. 9.7) to allow exerting traction on the upper and lower fragments until the two parts can be locked

Fig. 9.6 Holes made in
the upper and lower
portions of the sternum
using a drill to facilitate
later the placement of steel
wires that will approximate
the two fragments

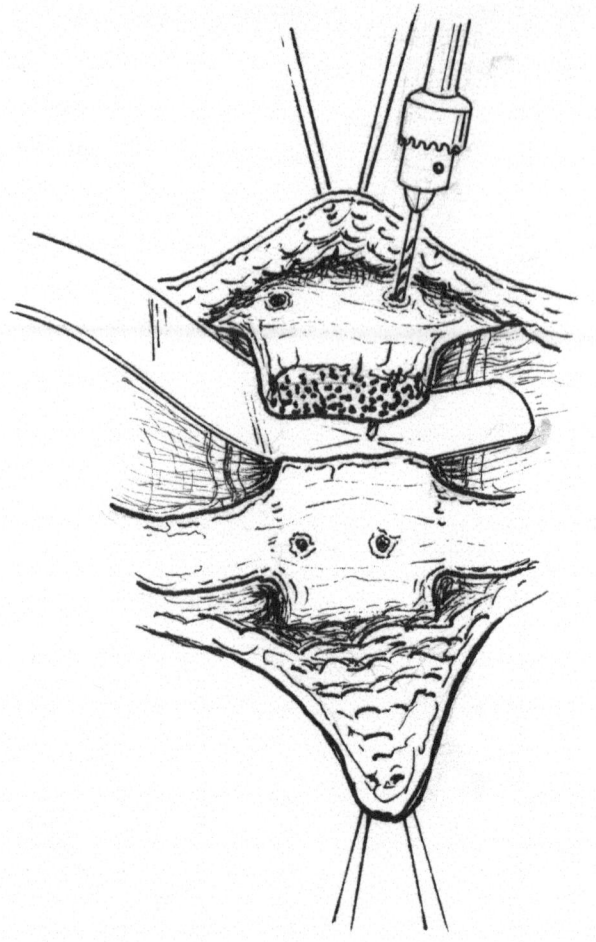

into place. This is greatly improved by creating a groove in the lower fragment and
also a wedge shape of the upper fragment. A standard narrow osteotome is very
effective to chisel the edges of the sternal fragments for this maneuver.

Stainless steel heavy-wire sutures are passed through the previously made holes
in both fragments (Fig. 9.8) but should not be tied together as yet. Use only wires
gauge 6 or 8 depending on the size of the patient.

Once the two fragments are locked into place, the wires are tied firmly
together.

In order to prevent lateral displacement of the fragments two stainless steel pins
are placed within the thickness of the bone, parallel to each other inserted from the
bottom up (Fig. 9.8). This is another reason why the hyperextension position of the
operating table is necessary to facilitate this step of the repair. Also the length of the

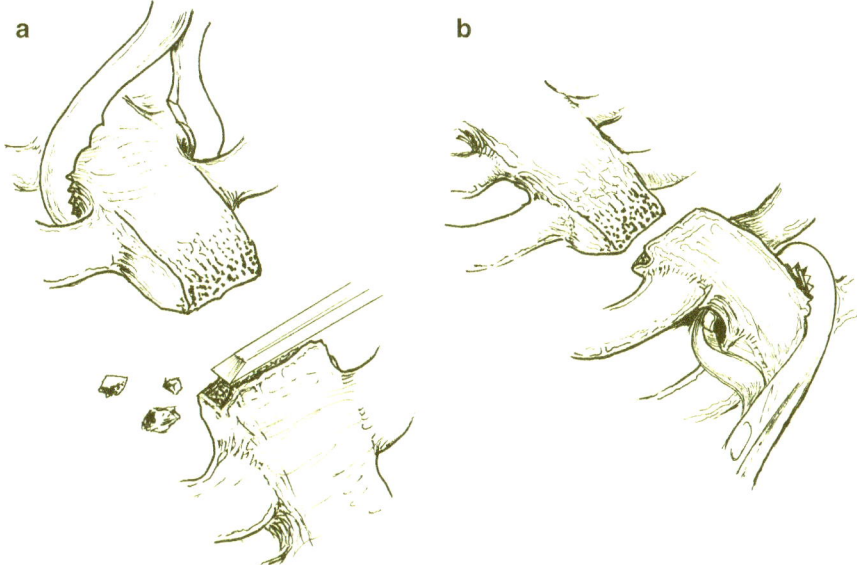

Fig. 9.7 (**a**, **b**) Large bone graspers are needed to manipulate the fractured segments of the sternum. Osteotome is used to chisel the edges of the fragments on both ends. The upper end is made a wedge and the lower portion is given a groove that facilitates locking of both fragments

Fig. 9.8 Heavy steel wires are placed in the perforated holes of the sternum and tied together. In addition to preventing lateral motion of the fragments, two Steinmann rods are placed lengthwise within the thickness of the bone from the bottom up (see text)

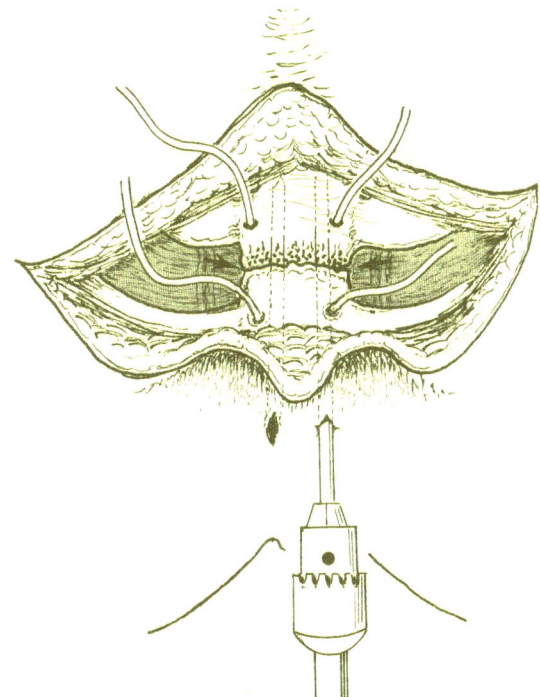

pins needs to be measured accurately and it is very helpful to have an extra pin freely laid just over the sternum to estimate at least one-and-a-half inch of the pin to be advanced into the upper bone fragment. It is very important to use only Steinmann **threaded** pins (3/32 or 1/16 in. in diameter) and not plain type to prevent migration of the pins, particularly at the lower end.

Postoperative radiograph should be obtained to verify the correct position of the Steinmann pins (Fig. 9.9).

Repair of the sternal fracture is complete. The wire sutures are tightened and the cut ends buried in the soft deep tissues. The Steinmann pins are cut flush to the bone (Fig. 9.10).

Placement of the wires in a figure-of-eight fashion may also work (Fig. 9.11) but may be more cumbersome to place and difficult to assure its tightness because of the stiffness of the wire of this caliber (Fig. 9.12) that does not slide easily like a regular suture.

In this operation the pleural cavities are not entered but at the end subcutaneous drains should be laid under the skin flaps.

In the follow-up period if any Steinmann pin migrates, it should be removed from below. No problems have been seen in the evolution of these patients.

Reference

1. J Thorac Cardiovasc Surg. 2005;130:445–448.

Fig. 9.9 View of the complete repair

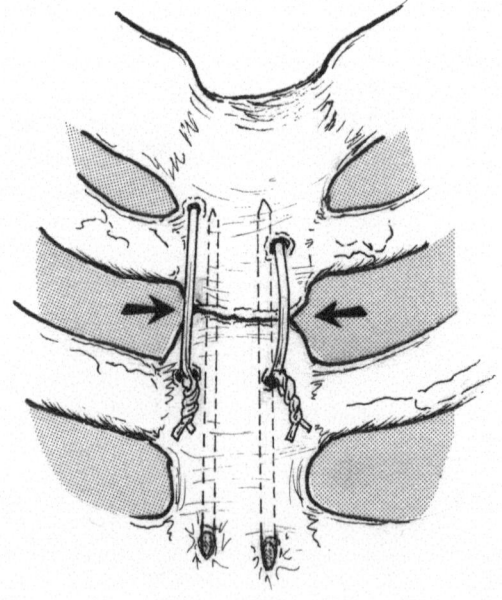

Fig. 9.10 Cross section
showing the rod position

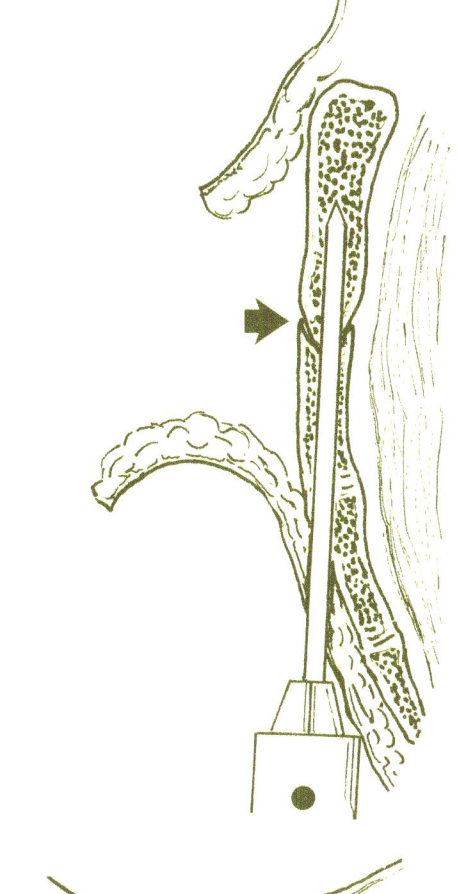

Fig. 9.11 Another option
to place the wires (see text)

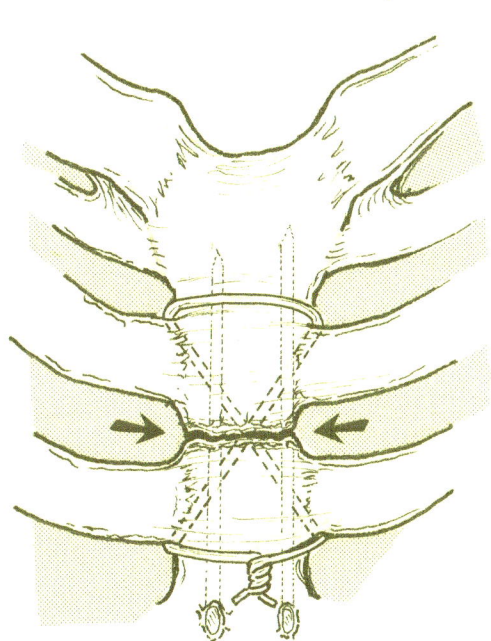

Fig. 9.12 Postoperative
radiography that shows the
position of the Steinmann
pins

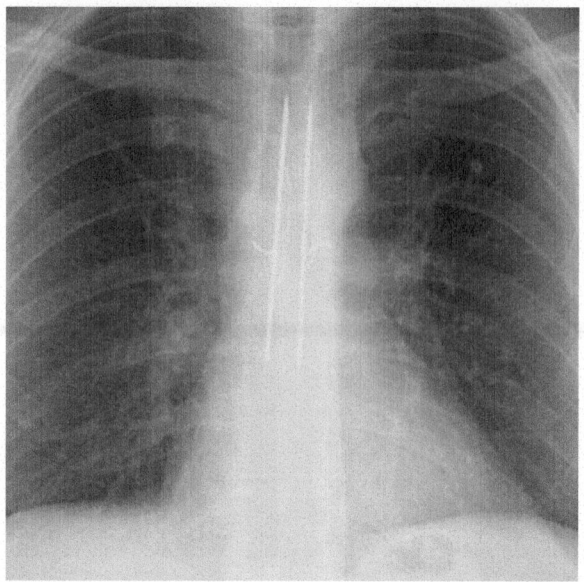

Part III
Cardiac Surgery Procedures and Techniques

Chapter 10
Pericardial Effusions and Cardiac Tamponade

Abnormal collection of fluid in the pericardial sack may occur in a wide variety of conditions. It may appear as a primary spontaneous pericarditis; in pulmonary infections; and as a sequel following a myocardial infarction. It may appear also due to undetected or late perforation of the right ventricular apex following implants of intravenous pacemaker or defibrillator leads; due to direct trauma to the chest; or as a late complication of a cardiac operation with or without the use of extracorporeal circulation particularly if the patient is on chronic anticoagulation regimen. It may occur also in the postoperative period after thoracic surgical intervention when the chest tubes are removed too soon when the drainage has not totally stopped. It may also develop in cases of a primary or metastatic malignant process.

The pericardial effusion may develop gradually but on occasions it presents with a rapid evolution. When suspected, the diagnosis is made by radiographic technique or more precisely by 2D echo exam. The correct treatment is to proceed with immediate evacuation of the fluid. Although placing a catheter percutaneously in the pericardial sack guided by ultrasound technique may be attempted, in most instances the effusion recurs or the evacuation of the pericardial content is not totally attained satisfactorily. That is the case when in addition to fluid the pericardium may contain blood clots that require a more complete effective drainage.

Therefore the correct treatment commonly requires a surgical intervention. In the case of chronic recurring effusion one technique that was used for many years is to construct what has been called a "pericardial window." This means to perform a thoracotomy, usually on the left side, with the obvious disadvantages of such procedures, some of which are mentioned here.

To create the so-called pericardial window requires the chest cavity to be entered in order to reach the pericardium. Any thoracotomy carries a painful postoperative course. There is a need to spread the ribs or even remove part of them. The phrenic nerve needs to be isolated and a portion of the pericardium is excised to allow a permanent drainage opening into the pleural cavity. Bleeding is always a possibility caused from the chest wall structures as well. In addition, if the pericardial effusion is causing pericardial tamponade with severe cardiac and respiratory compromise

© Springer International Publishing AG, part of Springer Nature 2018   49
J. E. Molina, *Cardiothoracic Surgical Procedures and Techniques*,
https://doi.org/10.1007/978-3-319-75892-3_10

the patient may become hemodynamically unstable. For this operation the patient needs to be positioned in lateral or semi-lateral position for the thoracotomy approach. This is not tolerated in a patient with already circulatory instability. This approach therefore must not be used and should be avoided whenever pericardial tamponade exists or is suspected. It is here therefore recommended that the most optimal and safer intervention is strongly what is here named "trans-xiphoid peri-cardiostomy" approach. In some textbooks it is addressed as "subxiphoid" but this is incorrect because the operation does not make a route under the xiphoid process but through it in order to provide for a better and safer operation. A description follows here:

A short vertical incision is made in the upper midline of the epigastrium from the base of the xiphoid process down for approximately of 23 in., depending on the patient's size and built (Fig. 10.1). In an obese patient the incision must be of adequate length to reach the midline. The incision enters the subcutaneous tissue until the xiphoid is exposed. The linea alba is incised gently being very careful not to enter the peritoneum. The xiphoid is lifted and dissected all the way around to clear the posterior surface up to the level of the sternum.

The xiphoid is split lengthwise and each half totally excised to its base (Fig. 9.4). A retractor is placed to keep the two sides of the incision spread. Now with blunt dissection the pre-peritoneal adipose and connective tissue are retracted down using

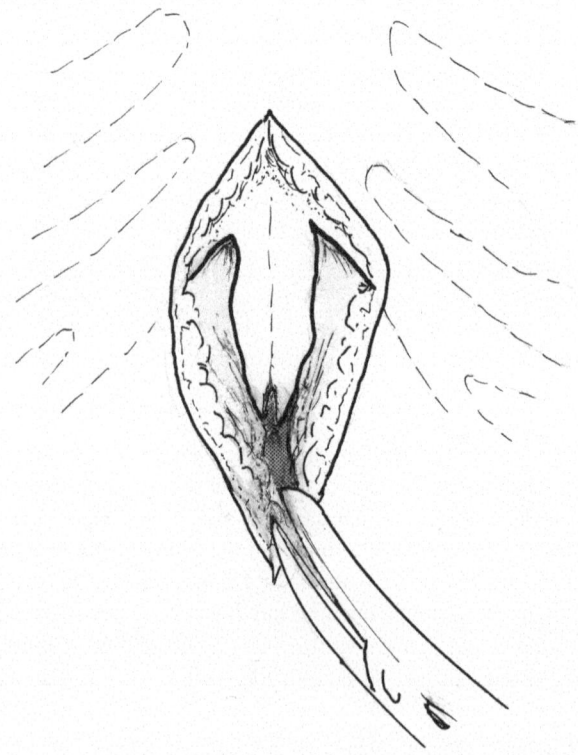

Fig. 10.1 Midline incision and splitting of the xiphoid process followed by its resection

Fig. 10.2 After excision of the xiphoid process, blunt dissection of the soft tissues with down traction is helpful to expose the pericardial sac in the upper end

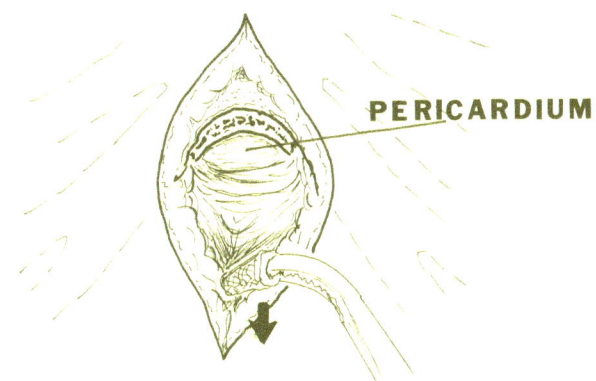

PERICARDIUM

a Kütner or a "peanut" forceps instrument (Fig. 10.2) until the substernal portion of the pericardium can be visualized. With digital exploration the pericardial sack is identified and the heart pulsations can be felt. Now the pericardium can be grasped, either with an instrument or, preferably, by placing a suture to exert traction, and with the cautery or scissors the pericardium is incised transversally (Fig. 10.3). Immediately the fluid pours out, most of the time under pressure. As soon as this is accomplished, the patient's blood pressure returns to normal and his/her cardiac rhythm stabilizes. A sample of pericardium should be obtained for pathology exam. A digital exploration of the pericardial cavity is carried out and removal of blood clots can be accomplished easily. Finally a soft pliable chest tube is inserted, secured to the skin, and connected to a drainage container. This operation takes a few minutes and with the patient in the supine position it is well tolerated.

The midline incision is now suture-closed in a routine manner.

Acute emergency situations of cardiac tamponade arise when a perforation or rupture of an intrapericardial organ is injured or perforated. A perforation of a coronary artery during a procedure being conducted by the cardiologist being this a dilation or implant of endovascular stent triggers an acute emergency situation that requires to be operated immediately. Trying to evacuate the blood percutaneously with a catheter is pointless and totally ineffective. The patient must be transferred to the surgical suite and operated.

In these cases there is no time for procrastination or to request diagnostic tests because the patient deteriorates in a matter of minutes. Therefore the "trans-xiphoid" operation described above is not applicable to that situation. Instead the patient requires an emergency sternotomy to stop the hemorrhage and to repair the inflicted damage to save the patient's life.

Reference

1. Pace. 1996;19:288–29.

Fig. 10.3 Incision of the
pericardium and drainage
of the pericardial fluid

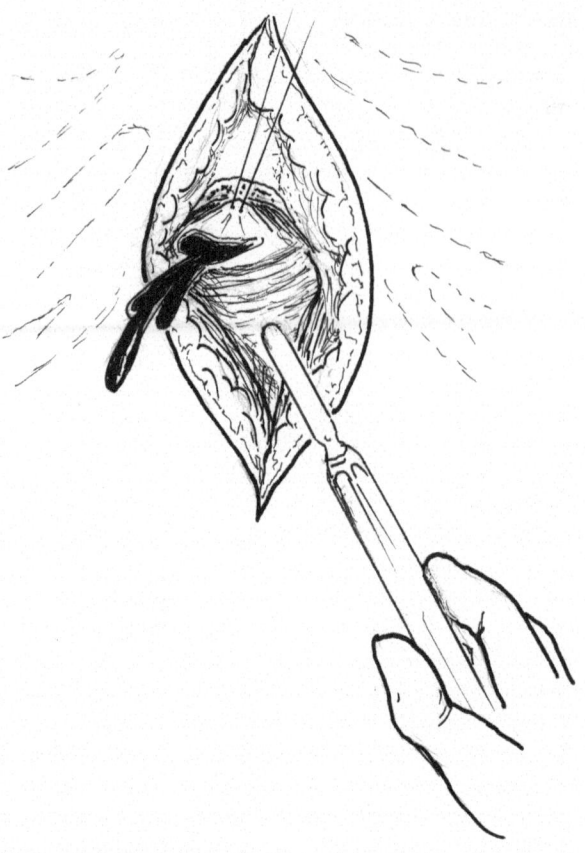

Chapter 11
The Use of Non-reversed Saphenous Veins

Harvested saphenous veins have been used as free vascular grafts in all areas of the human body as a substitute of arterial grafts to bridge a gap of absent circulation. The most frequent use of vein has been the performance of aortocoronary bypass operations. Despite the increased use of the internal thoracic arteries (mammary vessels) bilaterally, 70% of the grafts in these operations are still constituted by harvested saphenous veins. Also these veins are used for revascularization of the extremities, for carotid artery-intracranial bypass, repair of thoracic outlet veins, and also intra-abdominal vascular procedures. Current statistics indicate that saphenous veins harvested from the thigh have better patency rate than veins harvested from the legs. In addition, surgeons utilize and implant these veins in a reversed fashion to overcome the presence of the vein valves. Rheologically and kinetically this is a wrong concept because the blood in a vessel runs from the greater diameter toward the smaller end. Based on this concept to achieve a more logic setting, the use of non-reversed saphenous vein has been introduced to improve the flow mechanics and the durability of the bypass grafts. There are several devices designed for eliminating the valves of the vein to render it patent in its entire length. A simple metal valvulotome is provided with a blunt hook at the end but containing a cutting edge in its inferior curvature that only cuts on the way out when extracted.

There are other advantages to the use of non-reversed saphenous veins when harvested from the thigh instead of the leg: The normal bifurcations of the saphenous vein can be preserved and the two or even three branches can be connected to the recipient vessels with one single anastomosis to the aorta. Harvesting the vein from the thigh is also better tolerated by the patient because as long as the incision does not go below the knee level, no leg or foot edema develops and the thigh incisions heal better than cuts in the leg. In women this is a very important consideration.

© Springer International Publishing AG, part of Springer Nature 2018   53
J. E. Molina, *Cardiothoracic Surgical Procedures and Techniques*,
https://doi.org/10.1007/978-3-319-75892-3_11

Fig. 11.1 Dimensions of a
thigh harvested saphenous
vein. Proximal femoral end
of the vein measures 7 mm
and the distal end 4 mm.
Cross-sectional areas
indicated at those levels

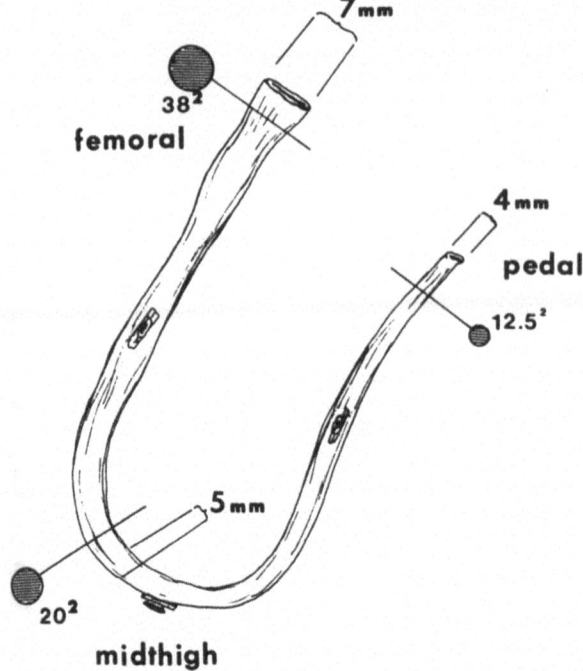

The adjunct illustration (Fig. 11.1) shows the normal dimensions of a thigh harvested saphenous vein from the groin down to above the knee level. The proximal or femoral end measures 7 mm in width. The midportion measures 5 and 4 mm in its distal end. The cross-sectional area measures in corresponding metric parameters are 38.2, 20.2, and 12.5 mm^2.

A blunt olive-tip metal needle is secured to the proximal femoral end of the vein (Fig. 11.2), and by gentle injection using a syringe with the chosen solution the vein is distended to the first valve. Simultaneously the metal valvulotome is introduced via the distal end (Fig. 11.3) and advanced to the level of the valve (Fig. 11.4). Then, pulling back the valvulotome the venous valve is severed making the vein patent to the level of the next valve. Gentle injection with the syringe will show the level of the next valve. In this manner the entire vein is now usable. Side smaller branches are obliterated with clips. The vein is now ready to be used. The forked branches of the main saphenous when used for additional bypass to other coronaries are handled in the same manner (Fig. 11.5); therefore we have now two grafts that can be anastomosed to the designed vessels with only one proximal end. Consequently only one proximal anastomosis is needed.

Fig. 11.2 Preparation of the vein by distending it by injecting from the femoral end. A metal valvulotome advanced from the distal end cuts the vein valves as the instrument is pulled back

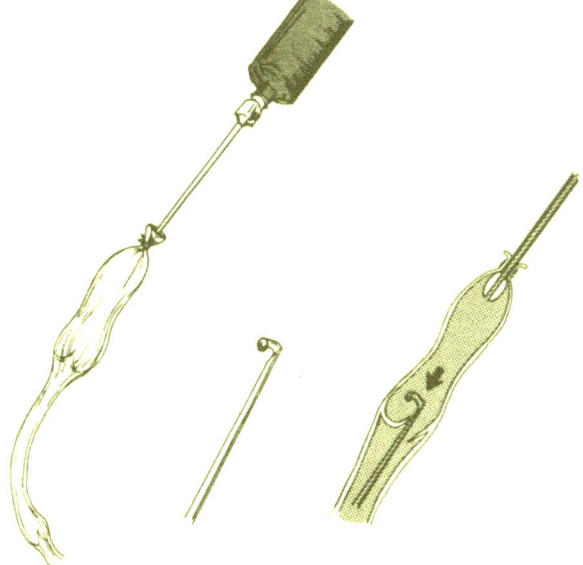

Fig. 11.3 A saphenous vein partially ready to be used

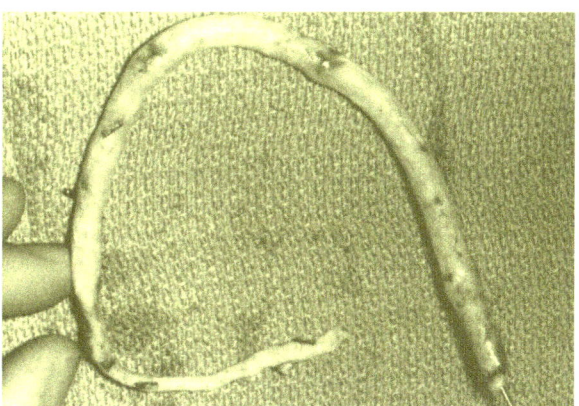

Fig. 11.4 Inserting the valvulotome in the vein distal end

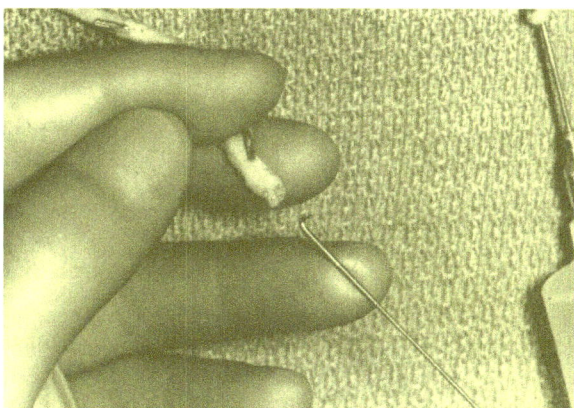

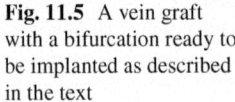

Fig. 11.5 A vein graft
with a bifurcation ready to
be implanted as described
in the text

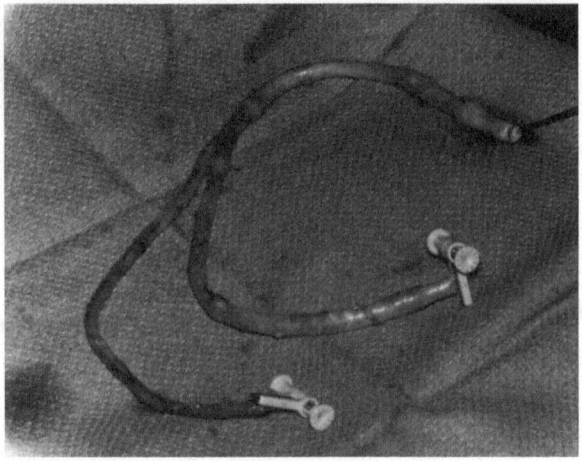

During the follow-up of the patient if a repeated angiogram is required, one single injection of contrast medium in the main graft will show all the distal connections. In our institution this technique has been used in over thousand cases without any problems and satisfactory long-term results.

References

1. Ann Thorac Surg. 1989; 48:624–7.
2. J Thorac Cardiovasc Surg. 1988; 36: 44–45.

Chapter 12
Patching of the Left Main Coronary Artery

The condition of left main coronary obstruction represents a very serious and risk situation for sudden death because it affects the circulation for the entire heart. If occlusion happens the patient dies instantly. Therefore the patients diagnosed with this finding are operated immediately after the diagnosis is made.

Direct opening of the obstruction is rarely undertaken by percutaneous intervention with balloon dilation and implant of stents. This is only attempted when the patient already has functioning patent bypass grafts in the distal vessels; therefore the intervention is considered a protected procedure.

Surgical direct widening of the main trunk is theoretically advantageous over multiple bypass grafts to the distal branches, because in addition the circulation to the heart is reestablished in a normal antegrade circulation fashion to a large portion of the myocardium in opposition to retrograde circulation by grafts of unknown durability.

Patching of the main coronary artery is a procedure rarely done because the great majority of patients with left main obstruction have distal obstruction of the terminal branches LAD, circumflex, and right coronaries. Therefore when surgical intervention is recommended to these patients, they are treated by placing independent bypass grafts in the distal vessels involved. In a study published in 2011, among 8720 patients with coronary disease, 5529 underwent coronary angiograms and left main obstruction was found in 468 (8.4%). The location of the obstruction is very important; thus only patients with ostial or midportion of the left main artery were considered candidates for direct surgical approach (Fig. 12.1). Among the 468 patients studied, only 16 had left main obstruction without identifiable left-sided distal obstructions, and in another 15 patients proximal right coronary disease was found in addition. Only 19 patients underwent the operation to be described here.

Not all patients undergoing left main patching were having first-time surgery. To illustrate this point three situations are described here: One 61-year-old woman had undergone internal mammary graft to the LAD and a saphenous vein graft to the circumflex. The left main had a 70% obstruction at the time. The circumflex graft

© Springer International Publishing AG, part of Springer Nature 2018
J. E. Molina, *Cardiothoracic Surgical Procedures and Techniques*,
https://doi.org/10.1007/978-3-319-75892-3_12

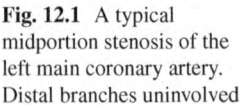

Fig. 12.1 A typical
midportion stenosis of the
left main coronary artery.
Distal branches uninvolved

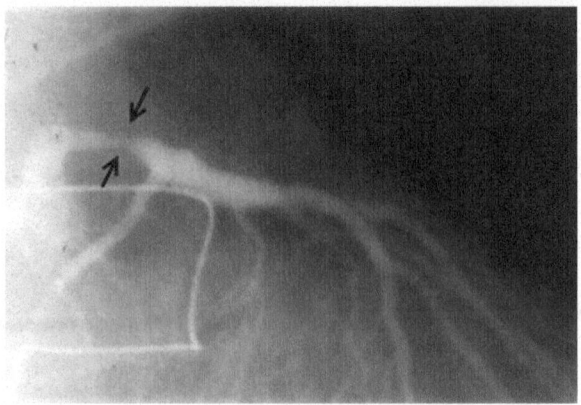

occluded 4 years later and she was very symptomatic. The left main obstruction
remained at 70%. Therefore at the time of her second operation a patch was placed
directly to the left main coronary and the mammary graft was left undisturbed. The
patient has done well for the following 11.5 years. A second patient had suffered
bacterial endocarditis developing mitral and aortic valve regurgitation. The left
main coronary had 80–90% obstruction. The patient underwent mitral and aortic
valve replacements and in addition the left main coronary was enlarged with a patch
of saphenous vein. The aortic prosthesis which was originally a tissue valve gradually showed deterioration and stenosis 2 years later requiring a second intervention
to replace the aortic valve prosthesis; this time a St. Jude valve prosthesis was
implanted and the patch to the left vein done 2 years earlier was found perfectly
healed and widely patent (Fig. 12.2). A third patient had been found to have a 90%
stenosis of the left main trunk and therefore she underwent a standard coronary
bypass operation both with saphenous veins to the distal LAD and to the obtuse
branch of the circumflex. However postoperatively she suffered cardiac arrest from
which she luckily recovered and survived. The patient refused further manipulations
and went home. However she continued having severe chest pain and she returned
for further evaluation. At this time, as suspected, the graft to the circumflex had
occluded and the vein graft to the LAD showed significant stenosis. The left main
again showed 90% stenosis. Accordingly she was reoperated and underwent directly
a patch to the left main without disturbing the other grafts. She had smooth recovery, and 10.5 years later she was still doing very well (Fig. 12.3).

These examples show that the obstruction of the left main should probably be
best treated with enlargement of the vessel if no other obstructions exist in the distal
circulation.

Among the group of patient treated in this manner there were two young women
who were diagnosed with Prinzmetal angina or spasm of the left main coronary who
presented a challenging diagnosis as well as therapeutic options. A coronary

Fig. 12.2 Angiogram
showing severe ostial
obstruction of the left main
coronary artery. The
contrast medium refluxes
into the Valsalva sinus

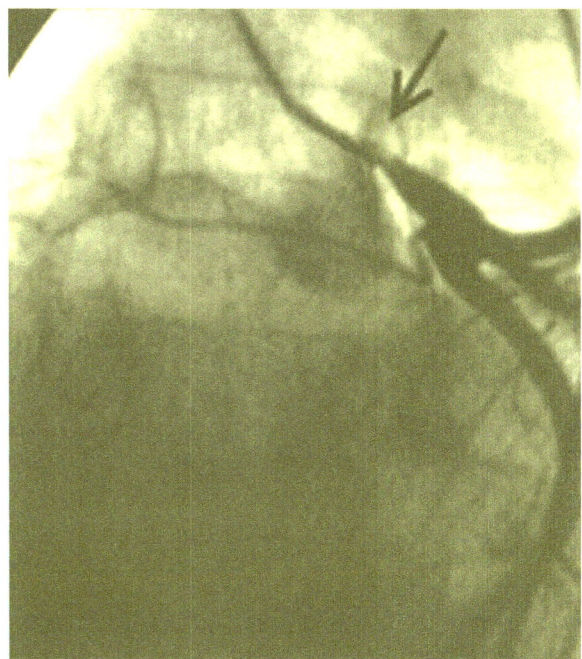

Fig. 12.3 Eleven years
postoperative angiogram
after left main patch
angioplasty. Patient
completely asymptomatic

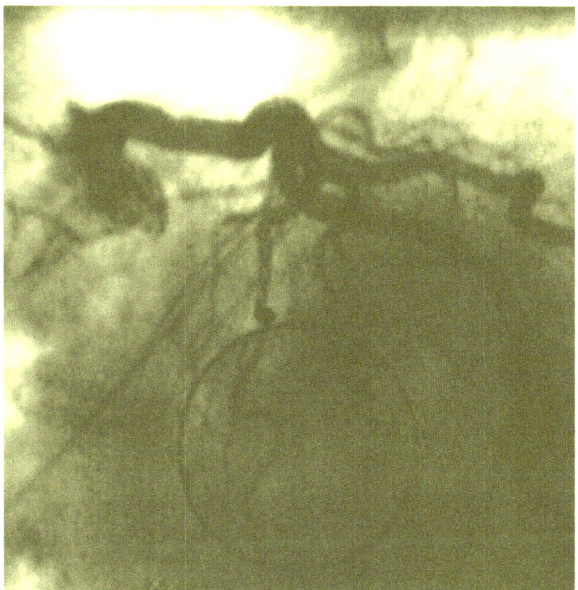

angiogram 2 months earlier had shown only 40% stenosis of the left main but the second angiogram was done now (which is 60 days later) because persistent symptoms showed a 70% obstruction with perfectly normal distal coronary arteries. These two patients were also treated with a left main patch and both had remained completely asymptomatic since.

Operative Procedure

The only patients showing left main obstruction recommended for this type of operation must have only ostial, proximal, or midportion of the artery involved and no obstruction toward the left main bifurcation. This group of patients constituted less than 8% of over 6000 patients with coronary disease.

To approach the left main trunk of the coronary arteries the root of the aorta must be exposed. The pulmonary artery must be retracted down in order to clearly visualize the origin of the left main artery. With the heart arrested and protected with cold retrograde cardioplegia, a transverse aortotomy is made at least 2 cm above the origin of the left main coronary. A piece of harvested saphenous vein or of pericardium readily available in the area is used to tailor a long patch.

Now from the aortotomy a vertical incision above the left main vessel is made and carried down to split the artery longitudinally from its origin to the distal end **without reaching the bifurcation** into the LAD and the circumflex (Fig. 12.4). This is one of the most important points to prevent any potential risk of narrowing any of these branches while laying the patch in place. The other important point is **do not do endarterectomy** of the left main vessel, particularly if it is calcified. Any

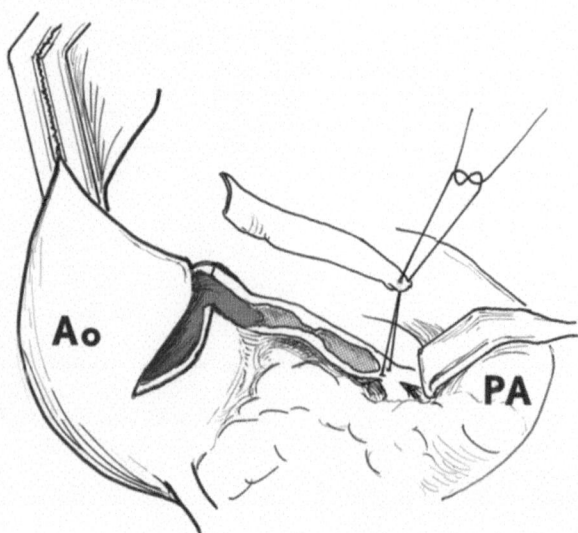

Fig. 12.4 Laying a saphenous vein patch over the split-opened left main coronary artery

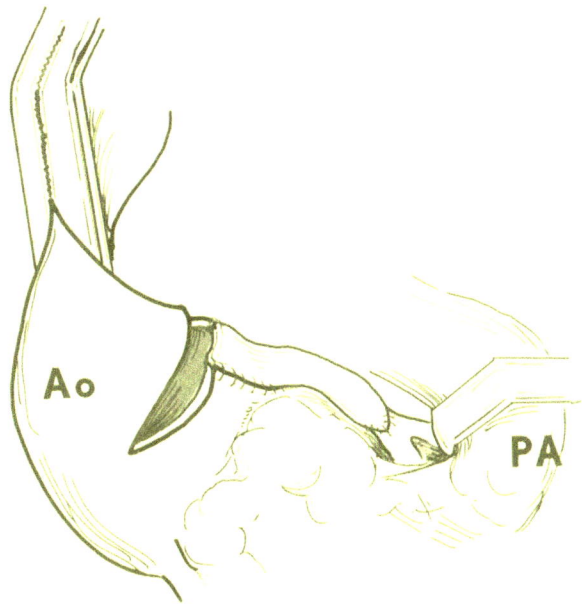

Fig. 12.5 Completed operation before closing the aortotomy

trauma to the endothelium of the coronary will lead to fibrosis and scar stenosis later on. Therefore very gently the vessel is split, and the venous patch previously tailored is brought into the field and sutured using fine monofilament suture material like 6-0 Prolene. The suture runs from the distal end in the coronary artery to the lip of the aortotomy incision (Fig. 12.5). Administering more retrograde cardioplegia the coronaries will fill retrograde verifying the patency of the graft. Now the aorta is closed with running everting suture using 4-0 Prolene. The air is vented out and the patient is gradually weaned off the cardiopulmonary bypass in the regular manner.

The follow-up after this operation has been gratifying when angiograms are done even years later for other reasons, showing good patency and no recurrence of the obstruction.

Coronary angiograms done in patients 10 1/2 and 12 years later have shown nicely wide open left main vessel and no aneurysmatic dilatation of the patch has been found.

Based on our experience treating these patients, when indicated, direct left main coronary widening patch is a good operation that the surgeons should be familiar with and should be performed more often.

Reference

1. Int J Angiol. 2011;20(3):143–147.

Chapter 13
Lymphocele After Vein Harvesting

Often enough after saphenous vein harvesting, regardless of the surgical method used, a lymphocele may develop in the upper thigh or even in the leg along the track of the vein site due to injury to the lymphatic channels. This complication is only apparent in the postoperative period usually after the patient has been discharged from the hospital. Simple needle puncture with syringe aspiration of the fluid does not solve the problem because as soon as the patient leaves the clinic the fluid begins collecting again. A more drastic procedure needs to be done, which could be easily conducted in the outpatient facility (Fig. 13.1).

Under local anesthesia a small incision is made in the upper part of the thigh, a few centimeters above and lateral to the end of the harvesting incision. A tunnel is created with a hemostatic forceps until it enters the pocket of fluid and a small drain can be inserted into the fluid collection. Usually a Jackson-Pratt size 14 is adequate (Fig. 9.2). This is connected to a compressible bulb to maintain continuous suction (Fig. 13.2).

Important points: Always make the incision above the upper end of the vein-harvested incision. This will allow the patient to carry the bulb pinned to his/her clothes or secured in any preferred manner. The patient needs to be instructed how to empty the suction bulb once or twice a day depending on the amount of drainage that collects. The drain size should be at least 14 or larger because otherwise a smaller drain tube may get clogged after a few days and then the drain must be replaced. The system works well and maintains the pocket collapsed. Once the drainage stops and there is no more evidence of a detectable pocket, the drain is removed. It may take up to 2 weeks or a few days longer for a large pocket to stop draining.

© Springer International Publishing AG, part of Springer Nature 2018   63
J. E. Molina, *Cardiothoracic Surgical Procedures and Techniques*,
https://doi.org/10.1007/978-3-319-75892-3_13

Fig. 13.1 Typical aspect
of a left thigh lymphocele
formed under the
vein-harvesting incision

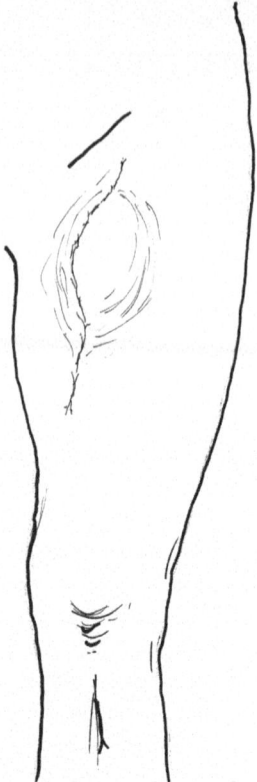

During that time the patient should be kept on prophylactic antibiotic therapy to prevent infection.

If infection develops in such incisions, which could be severe with erythema and edema, the treatment changes. The patient needs to be hospitalized. The treatment requires reopening of the entire incision, debridement, and placement of a drain system, but this time the wound needs to be cleansed up completely, removing all the previous suture material (usually absorbable). The wound must be irrigated with antibiotic solution. Do not use Betadine because it will impair the fibroblast repair progress and interferes with the white cell function. The incision must be closed with interrupted sutures in a single layer with a monofilament material like Prolene size 0 or 2 (Fig. 13.3). These sutures should stay until the wound is healed, and no drainage is produced. Total healing takes approximately from 12 days to 2 weeks. During that period antibiotic treatment must be implemented. Twice a day the incision should be cleansed with aseptic solution like Techni-Care, Hibiclens, or Betasept to prevent crust from forming under the sutures.

Fig. 13.2 Treatment of the
lymphocele by implanting
a drain connected to a
suction bulb

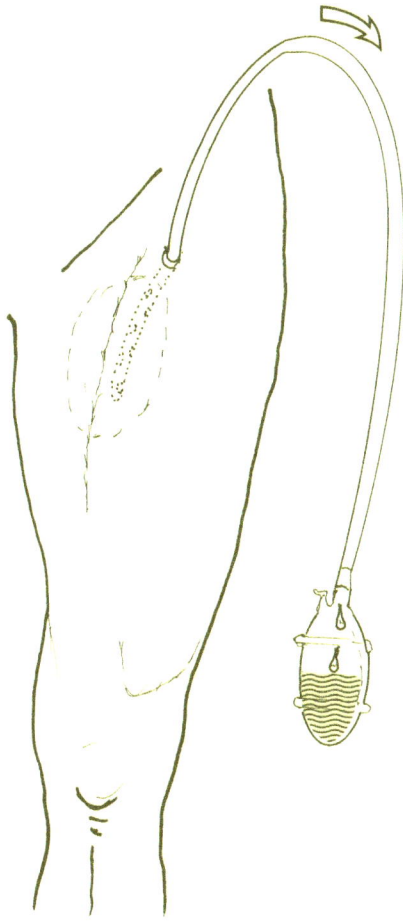

Fig. 13.3 If the entire
wound becomes infected,
the wound must be opened
and debrided and the
incision is closed as a
single layer with
interrupted size 2-0 or size
0 Prolene sutures in
addition to implanting a
drain under suction (see
text)

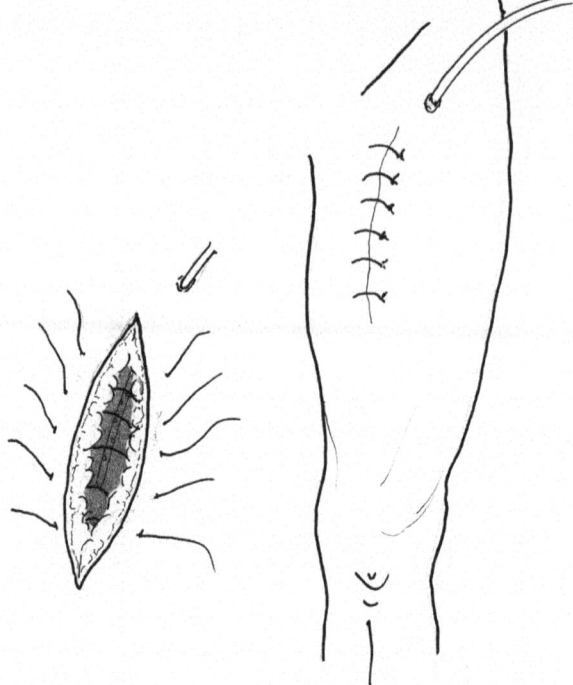

Chapter 14
Placement of Temporary Epicardial Pacer Leads

Currently, there is no discussion about the benefits of implanting temporary pacemaker leads in the heart following any type of open cardiac surgical operation. The advantages are multiple including the treatment of severe bradycardia or any type of cardiac atrioventricular block, as well as diagnosis of cardiac arrhythmias. Therefore the placement of temporary wires is routinely done regardless of the cardiac corrective operation undertaken. However, in the past, the primary reason for placing a temporary pacing lead was to pace the ventricle if complete heart block had occurred. We know now that pacing the ventricle alone is not a satisfactory approach to increase the cardiac output because the heart does not retain its normal atrioventricular sequential rhythm, and actually in many occasions ventricular pacing alone makes the situation worse causing hypotension.

The proper manner to stabilize the cardiac rate and rhythm conduced to increase the cardiac output is to electrically pace the atrium and if the A-V conduction is delayed the ventricle is paced synchronically as well.

After open-heart surgery the elderly patient in particular shows bradycardia after discontinuing the cardiopulmonary bypass. Rates of 50–70 are commonly seen in part because of the medications (beta-blockers most commonly) that the patient had been taking before he/she came to surgery.

Since temporary pacemaker leads should be routinely implanted, the decision should be made on the type of leads and their optimal position as well as whether a unipolar type of pacing will be sufficient or a bipolar type would be preferable.

In this chapter it is explained why a bipolar should always be used because with the unipolar system when the electrical current is delivered to the electrode in the heart, the other ground electrode is usually placed in the subcutaneous tissue to establish the electrical circuit. This causes uncomfortable irritation at the skin level particularly in children where this situation becomes intolerable and therefore unacceptable. A bipolar system does not have such disadvantages.

The time, during the course of the operation, when the electrons should be placed is important for a smooth process and clean surgical maneuver.

© Springer International Publishing AG, part of Springer Nature 2018   67
J. E. Molina, *Cardiothoracic Surgical Procedures and Techniques*,
https://doi.org/10.1007/978-3-319-75892-3_14

When the patient's corrective operation has been completed and rewarming is started it is the perfect time to implant the electrodes. At that point the heart is totally decompressed still on bypass and the heart can be easily manipulated. First the atrial pacer bipolar system is implanted. The best site is in the posterior wall of the atrium. The atrial cannulas are deflected toward the left side. This maneuver exposes the atrial posterior wall and the interatrial groove. The lead system is implanted by using the bipolar Medtronic model 6500 which consists of a silicon disc (Fig. 14.1) with perforations on opposite sides for the sutures to be placed that will hold the disc against the atrial wall. Two wire electrodes are passed along the central portion of the disc making sure to keep the metal bead in the center of the disc which will be in contact with the atrial wall (Fig. 14.2). The rest of the electrode lead ahead of the metal bead consists of a coiled Prolene 4-0 suture which holds the electrodes in place. The electrodes must be threaded in the disc before attaching the disc to the atrium. A 5-0 suture is placed parallel to the interatrial groove. This is passed through the orifices in the disc to be tied later. A second similar suture is placed in front of the first one and also passed through the opposite edge of the disc. Both sutures are now tied bringing the electrodes against the wall of the atrium. The patient is weaned off the cardiopulmonary bypass and the electrodes are laid along the lateral surface of the heart and brought through the abdominal wall to the outside securing them to the skin to prevent dislodgment. The electrodes may be connected to the external pacing unit any time (Fig. 14.3). Placing the atrial pacing wires in the back has the advantage of having the heart laying on them favoring better contact with the heart.

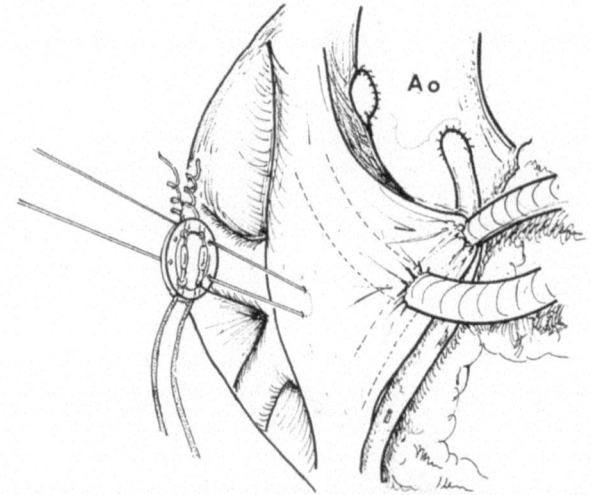

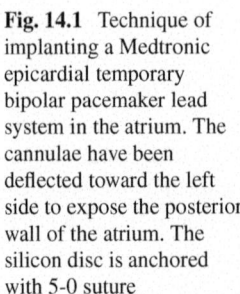

Fig. 14.1 Technique of implanting a Medtronic epicardial temporary bipolar pacemaker lead system in the atrium. The cannulae have been deflected toward the left side to expose the posterior wall of the atrium. The silicon disc is anchored with 5-0 suture

Fig. 14.2 A second suture secures the disc containing the two temporary leads in contact to the atrial wall

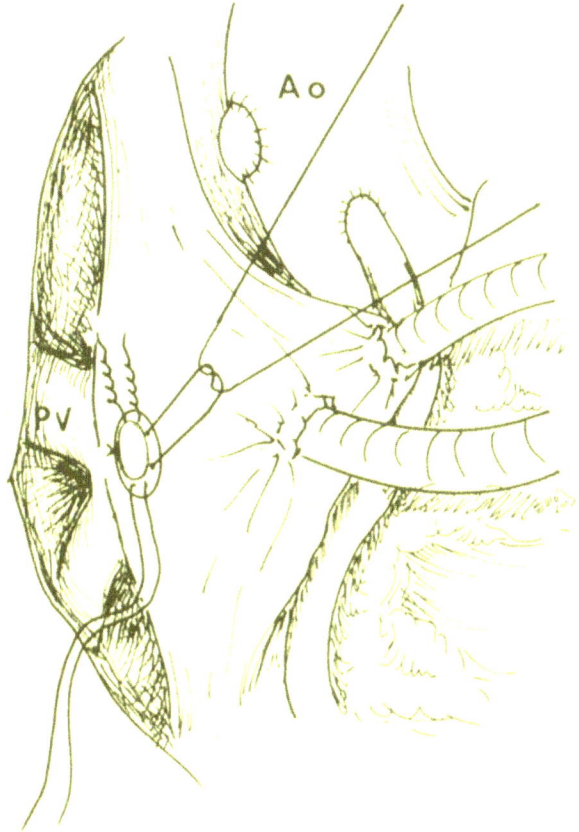

The atrial wall is thicker in the back and very thin in the front. In children particularly placing atrial electrodes should be done preferably in the posterior wall while the patient is still on bypass and the atrium decompressed, not in the front. If the electrodes are placed on the anterior surface of the atrium they often bleed and if the bare wires are stitched to the atrium their removal may cause bleeding or they can't be removed without taking the patient back to surgery.

Placement of the ventricular electrode is simply done by anchoring it to an avascular area in the anterior wall of the right ventricle. This could be accomplished after the patient is off cardiopulmonary bypass and decannulated. After eliminating the needle of the electrode, the coiled portion of the lead keeps it in place. There is no need to place additional holding sutures.

Fig. 14.3 The leads are now laid under the heart passed to the exterior through the abdominal wall. Secured with a skin stitch

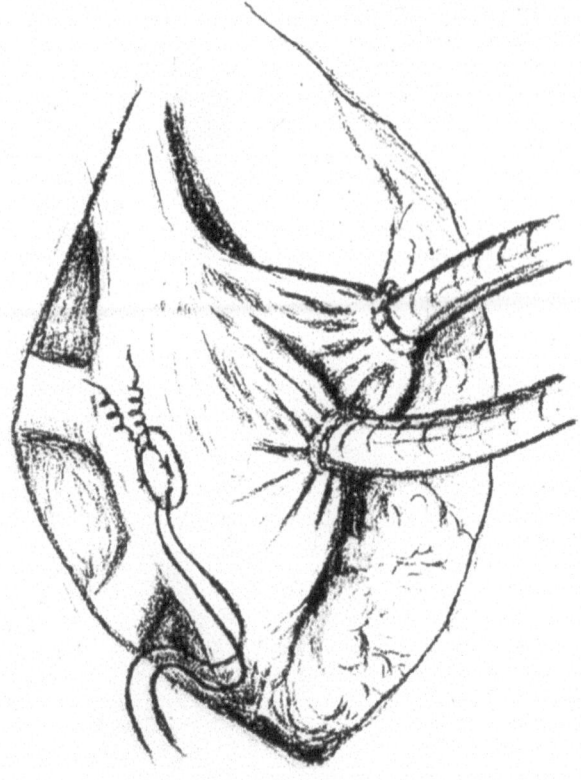

The parameters to pace the heart are as follows: After surgery if the spontaneous rate is between 50 and 70, it is preferable to pace the atrium at the rate of 90 beats per minute. This maneuver increases the cardiac output and helps to have the patient eliminate the third-space fluid accumulated in the tissues from the use of extracorporeal circulation. Usually pacing of the heart is implemented from 8 to 12 h. It could extend to 24 h until the patient recovers his/her normal usual adequate heart rate.

Removal of the electrodes is simply accomplished by exerting gentle but steady traction until they dislodge.

References

1. Medtronic News. Spring 1989:24–28.
2. J Thorac Cardiovasc Surg. 1983;85:625.

Chapter 15
Tricuspid Valve Replacement in Patients with Functioning Transvenous Pacemaker Lead

Replacement of the tricuspid valve is an operation not done frequently and the reports in the literature have shown a higher mortality than other valve replacements like mitral or aortic. This often attends to the multiple factors that lead to that event. Almost all patients that are referred for tricuspid valve replacement have undergone several or many prior cardiac operations. Frequently, this has happened as a result of the long-term evolution of congenital cardiac malformations like tetralogy of Fallot, transposition of the great vessels, Ebstein malformation, and others. Many of these patients survive to adulthood thanks to the pervious operations undertaken in their childhood, adolescence, or younger years. The presence of these anomalies is associated commonly with cardiac arrhythmias and most prominently with heart block. Consequently the patients often have already a pacemaker lead in place implanted intravenously in the right ventricle.

When the tricuspid valve develops severe regurgitation and needs to be replaced, a frequent practice seen in the past had been that at the time of the tricuspid valve replacement, the surgeon also proceeds to remove the pacing lead from the ventricle and provides the patients with an epicardial system. This practice is no longer justi-fied for several reasons; one of them is that there is overwhelming evidence that the intravenous pacemaker leads have better performance and durability than the epi-cardial counterparts. Also with a new lead a new tunnel must also be created to reach the site of the pulse generator and, in addition, the pocket containing the pacer pulse generator must be opened exposing the patient to a risk for infection.

To avoid these potential problems a functioning intravenous pacer lead in the right ventricle should be left in place without interfering with the process of the tricuspid valve replacement.

This conservative technique had been reported since 2004 but no publications appeared until our experience reported in 2010 with the use of the St. Jude valve prosthesis in that position. The durability and the functional parameters of the pace-maker lead left undisturbed have remained stable and unchanged during the long term of follow-up period from 9 to 12 years.

© Springer International Publishing AG, part of Springer Nature 2018
J. E. Molina, *Cardiothoracic Surgical Procedures and Techniques*,
https://doi.org/10.1007/978-3-319-75892-3_15

Technique of the Operation

After the right atrium is entered, the pacing lead is identified. In some cases the chronic lead is adherent along the inferior wall of the right ventricle; other times the lead is mostly free except for the tip of it firmly attached to the apex of the ventricle. In one case the lead when originally implanted had perforated one of the tricuspid leaflets causing the valve regurgitation. While conducting the tricuspid valve surgery the pacing lead is carefully dissected off the valve leaflets and the remaining valvular apparatus is removed. As the pledgeted sutures that will anchor the prosthetic valve to the annulus are placed in the posterior annulus (Fig. 15.1), the pacemaker lead is accommodated between two of them and the sutures on each side of the lead are passed through the skirt of the prosthesis without leaving any space between them. The pacing lead therefore is excluded from the valve operating mechanism and does not interfere with its function. When all the sutures are placed around the valvular annulus, the lead remains secured snugly between the normal valve tissue and the prosthetic cuff. The pacer lead should not be positioned between the arms of the suture that will be tied to secure the prosthesis.

Among the patients that have undergone this type of implant in our institution, there were patients with previous corrections for tetralogy of Fallot. One of them, a 42-year-old man, had suffered complete heart block at the time of a second

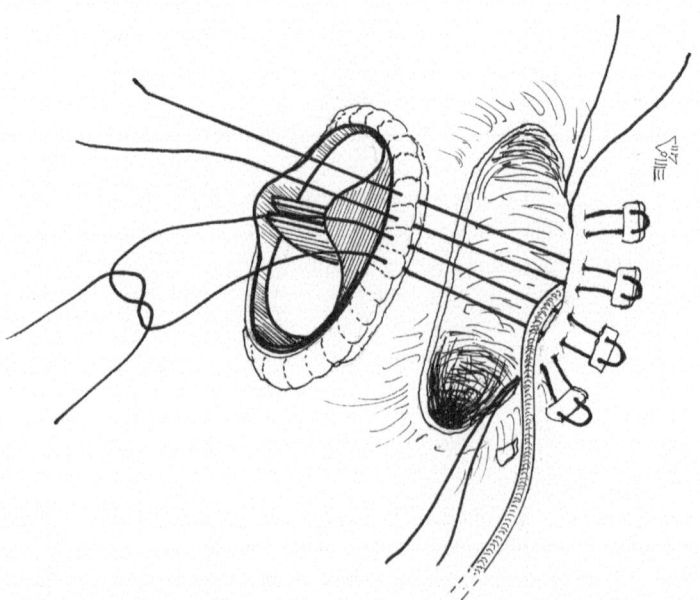

Fig. 15.1 Upon implanting the tricuspid valve prosthesis, the pacemaker lead is accommodated between two valve-holding stitches without interfering with the valve function mechanism

corrective operation and therefore had a pacemaker system implanted. Years later he developed severe aortic, pulmonary, and tricuspid regurgitation. At the time of his third operation the aortic, pulmonary, and tricuspid valves were replaced with St. Jude prosthetic valves. This patient is doing well as a college teacher 12 years later with a perfectly functioning pacemaker.

Another female patient 39 years old, also with tetralogy of Fallot, underwent mitral, pulmonary, and tricuspid valve replacement also with St. Jude prosthesis implementing the same operation, and has now a follow-up over 10 years. Two other patients with complex problems underwent this same operation and their survival is now approximating 9 and 10 years, respectively, all with the functioning pacemaker that has required replacements of the pulse generator but with still the same functioning lead.

This approach is therefore highly recommended and favored over removing the pacemaker lead to allow the implant of the prosthetic valve in the tricuspid orifice as long as the pacing parameters remain in the desired range.

The only questionable disadvantage is that when the need arises of replacing the pulse generator, this must be done by the surgeon to avoid any risk of infection of the pacing system which will be disastrous, because if this occurs the entire lead must be removed and if the infection reaches the intracardiac portion of the lead the tricuspid prosthetic valve would have to be removed as well. The sterility of an operating room suite is more strict than in a cardiac catheterization lab where the nurses and technical personnel walk in and out of the room frequently. The hallways outside of the catheterization labs also are not restricted to only scrub and masked personnel. Consequently, it is recommended that in cases that represent a very delicate condition like the one we have described in this section, it is preferable to have any intervention on the pacemaker system done in the operating room suite.

References

1. J Heart Valve Dis. 2004;13:523-4.
2. Ann Thorac Surg. 2010;89:318-2.

Chapter 16
Removal of Atrial Myxoma

The most common location where the myxoma tumor develops is in the cardiac atrial tissues, although this type of tumor has also been found in the ventricles and even in the great vessels particularly in the pulmonary artery confluence. Most of the time the tumor is of benign nature but rarely it can become malignant. However the main characteristic is the large size that may attain causing symptoms due to obstruction of flow through the mitral valve. In 80% of the cases the origin site is located in the left atrial septum near the mitral valve attached to the septum by a stalk involving the endocardium of the septum. The tumor is friable but covered by endothelium. Potentially it may lead to peripheral embolization in the arterial circulation. Since the tumor originates in the left atrium, the risk for embolism is real. Friability of this type of tumor has caused cerebral embolism and all organs in the peripheral arterial circulation are possible targets. The diagnosis of the tumor has been made after an embolus in the femoral artery was found to be myxoma.

The diagnosis is made usually by 2D echo ultrasound and less commonly by angiography. Once the diagnosis is made, surgery becomes the treatment of choice to remove it totally as safe as possible. Its removal therefore must be done very carefully to prevent fragmentation of the tumor. The operation requires extracorporeal circulation and an atriotomy to excise the tumor. In the past, most commonly the surgeon used to make a vertical incision in the back of the left atrium, past the interatrial septum. No digital manipulations are permitted to prevent braking of the friable tumor that may cause embolization. However this approach poses some limitations and it may risk incomplete resection due to limited exposure; thus the atrial incision may not provide large enough opening to deliver the tumor which sometimes is very large, or to clearly visualize the base of the stalk. This is so obvious in patients with small hearts or without dilated left atrium. To prevent these limitations and have a direct clear visualization of the base of the stalk enabling precise excision of the endocardium without damaging the tissues in the vicinity, a different approach was designed, namely a transseptal route as follows.

A double cannulation of the right atrium must be implemented (Fig. 16.1).

© Springer International Publishing AG, part of Springer Nature 2018

J. E. Molina, *Cardiothoracic Surgical Procedures and Techniques*,

https://doi.org/10.1007/978-3-319-75892-3_16

Fig. 16.1 After opening the right atrium the foramen ovale is identified and the incision begins at the highest point (see asterisk) and the incision is carried along the posterior and anterior insertions of the septum (S). *Ao* aorta

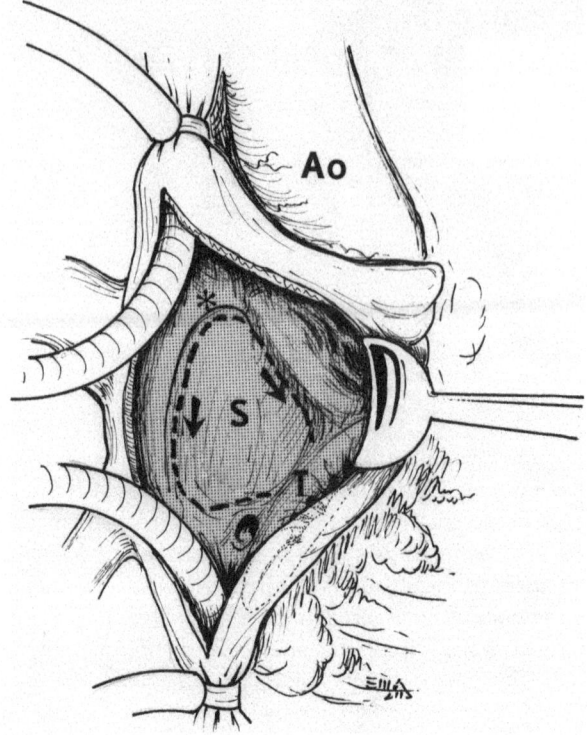

The right atrium is now entered through a generous incision. The foramen ovale is identified. An incision is made in the highest point and extended upwards toward the superior vena cava (see asterisk in Fig. 16.2). Then, the incision is extended along the interatrial septum anteriorly and posteriorly in a circumferential fashion creating a flap formed by the interatrial septum. Placing stitches in the edges of the septal flap for traction allows the entire tumor to be exposed and the base of the stalk can be easily visualized in the posterior ridge near the mitral valve annulus. A precise cut can be made around the base of the myxoma stalk. The traction to expose is exerted only on the interatrial septum, not on the tumor. Now safely the septum is removed along with the tumor attached to it. No manipulations are necessary and the risk of fragmenting the tumor is completely avoided. After verifying the complete excision of the tumor, the interatrial septum is replaced with a piece of prosthetic material or pericardium. Finally, the right atrium is closed and the operation terminated.

Reference

1. Thorac Cardiovasc Surgeon (Special Issue). 1990;38:183-191.

Fig. 16.2 A flap is
constituted by the septum
which is retracted exposing
the tumor down to the stalk
and excised without
disturbing the tumor. *Ao*
aorta, *M* mitral valve
orifice, *S* septum

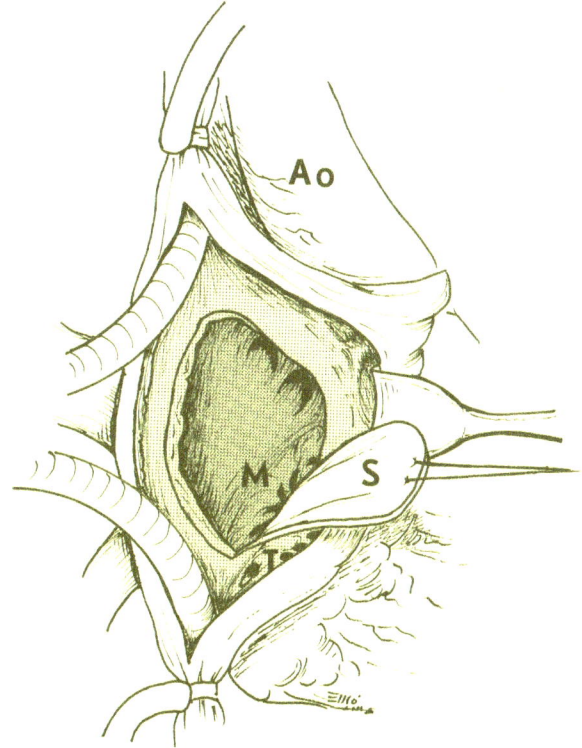

Chapter 17
Repair of Postoperative Sternal Wound Dehiscence with Mediastinitis

This is a major serious complication with significant rate of mortality and morbidity. Infection is almost always present and is not easy to treat. To attain cure in this situation requires a drastic approach and, as we know, only one surgical approach designed at our institution has rendered a 98% cure rate with no deaths.

Any cardiac operation done through a midline sternotomy potentially carries the risk of becoming dehisced caused by separation of the sternal bone, particularly in obese individuals, patients with osteoporosis, or simply large individuals who have the sternum closed without reinforcing the sides of the bone. The wire stitches holding the two halves of the sternum gradually may cut through the bone leading to eventual separation of the bone and also causing fracture at that level. Therefore in our experience, any patient with a body mass index (BMI) should receive reinforcement of the sternum closure as described in this section.

The dehiscence may occur as early as 7 days post-op, but 72% happen within 3 weeks. A few occur as late as 2 months. Therefore all patients undergoing midline sternotomy incisions should be thoroughly evaluated before they are operated and also before discharged to home; thus, the earlier the complication is detected, the easier the treatment may be to undertake.

As soon as the dehiscence is diagnosed the patient needs to be returned to the operating room for its repair and begin the effective treatment that requires 2 weeks of hospitalization. Since most of the patients have been found to have infection, the antibiotic treatment must be started immediately. The infective organism belongs most commonly to the Staphylococcus species.

The operation needed to repair the dehiscence is a tedious undertaking that may require up to four plus hours. Depending on how late the patient is brought for the repair so are the difficulties encountered in the operating suite, because the later the patient is returned for the repair the more likely the patient has developed more fractures of the sternum at the level where the previous wire stitches were placed. The complete treatment of this complication entails three very important stages:

© Springer International Publishing AG, part of Springer Nature 2018   79
J. E. Molina, *Cardiothoracic Surgical Procedures and Techniques*,
https://doi.org/10.1007/978-3-319-75892-3_17

The first one is the surgical procedure itself but the second just as important is the postoperative care which takes 2 weeks in the hospital. The third stage involves the late postoperative care.

Diagnosis

In obese individuals it is more difficult to diagnose the complication in the immediate postoperative period but some signs are helpful. One of them is observed when the patient continues complaining of incisional pain even after the third day. Normally the pain is well tolerated and practically is not an issue after the third day; however if it continues one must be alert to further investigate if possible dehiscence is developing. On occasions, the patient reports a grinding sensation with the arm movements or while rotating in bed. Palpation over the incision may help but is usually noncontributory in obese individuals due to the depth of the subcutaneous tissue. Radiographic studies are helpful but never plain views of the chest. To visualize the position of the sternal wires the proper study should be an overpenetrated view of the dorsal spine. This is the only plain study that may help to make the diagnosis. Otherwise a full CT scan of the chest is also definitely diagnostic. As soon as the presence of dehiscence is confirmed or strongly suspected, the patient must be returned to the operating suite for correction.

Stage 1: The Operation

The operative procedure is described first here:

Once the patient is fully anesthetized, the previous entire incision is rendered open and all the previously used suture material, absorbable or nonabsorbable without exception, must be removed to eliminate potential focus of recurring infection. All wire stitches must be removed as well regardless of their position holding the sternum. As soon as this is accomplished, the incision must be irrigated with antibiotic solution (usually cephalothin or cefamandole at 0.1% concentration) **always using a pressurized system** like the Davol device (Cranston, RI) with a splash guard. Do not use Betadine solution because it causes inhibition of the fibrous tissue for healing and interferes negatively with the white cell function in the presence of infection. If a large collection of purulent material is encountered as well as loose parts of fractured sternum the irrigation and debridement of fibrinous material are thoroughly undertaken but no bone is ever removed.

Now the first step is to dissect the soft-tissue layer on both sides of the incision by undermining the subcutaneous tissue with the skin, in one single layer. This is done with the cautery observing careful hemostasis (Fig. 17.1). This dissection is carried out laterally on both sides until the level of the intercostal spaces is reached

Fig. 17.1 Lateral dissection as a single layer of skin and subcutaneous tissue beyond the intercostal spaces

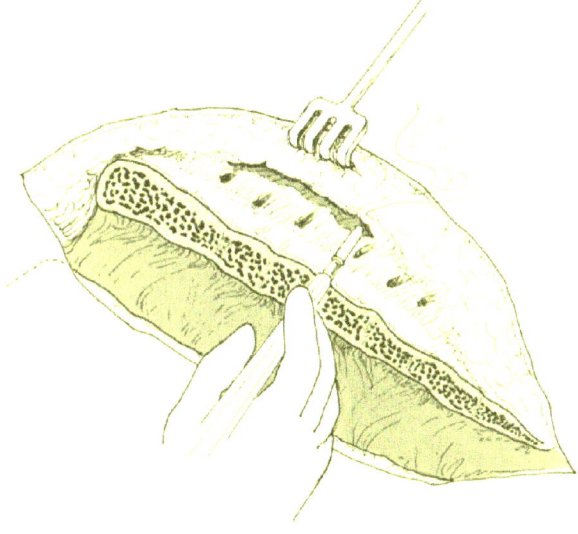

Fig. 17.2 Maneuver to assure that the single layer is sufficiently loose to be pulled pass the midline without any tension

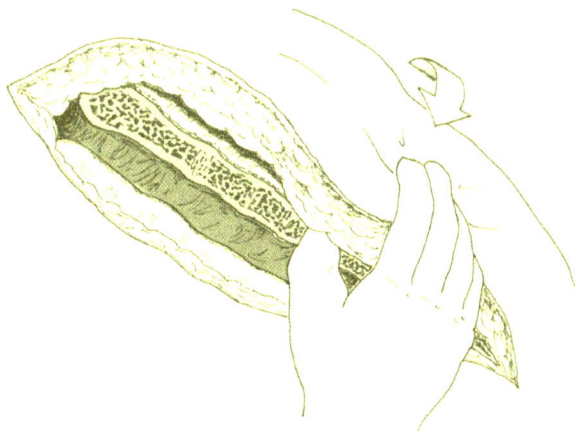

and passed. To assure that this layer is sufficiently loose to reach the midline at the end of the operation, the surgeon grabs the combined flap with gentle traction (Fig. 17.2) along the entire length of the incision. This maneuver is done on both sides of the sternum. Upon completion of this stage the wound is irrigated again as before with the same system. As a rule, the wound must be irrigated with the antibiotic solution after each stage of this operation.

The next stage is the more delicate part of the intervention. Retracting gently lifting the sternum on each side (a rake retractor works very well) the retrosternal space is dissected also using the cautery making sure to stay flush to the bone until the intercostal spaces are reached and passed laterally. Often enough the sternum

Fig. 17.3 A reinforcing wire suture gauge 8 is run along the lateral border of the sternum. Notice the drill bit that makes a hole in the manubrium in order to bring the reinforcing lateral suture up to that level (see text)

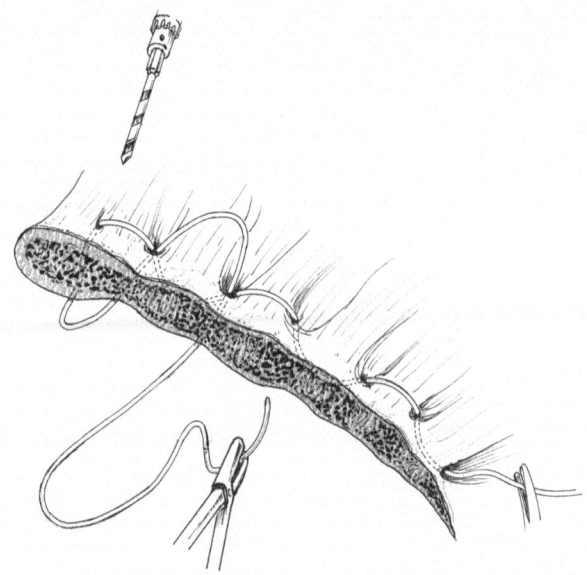

may show fractures caused by the previous wires placed at the original operation. The fractures are produced by the wires cutting through the bone which is the reason the sternum dehisces. The number of fractures varies from one to four on each side. This makes the dissection difficult but the fragments of the sternum must be left in place. No sternal bone is removed even if it looks loose. Once the dissection is completed on both sides, the most risky part of the operation is over. Again irrigation is done again after each stage.

The sternal repair is undertaken. Using heavy wire gauge 8 single long strand, 30 long provided with a blunt-end needle (A&E Medical Corp., Durham, NC) is required because the wire suture goes up and down along around each rib the entire length of the sternum. Starting at the lower end at the base of the xiphoid process, the suture goes lacing it around each rib flush to the sternum up to the manubrium and returns in reverse manner to the end of the sternum (Fig. 17.3). In the manubrium a hole must be made using a drill in order to have this parallel reinforcing suture above the first intercostal space. This will allow the placement of the next layer of sutures that will bring the two halves of the sternum together all the way up to the manubrium level. The single long-strand wire suture as described must be placed very snugly around each rib. This is very important to attain a perfect repair. Once the two ends of the reinforcing wire meet at the lower end, they are twisted the usual way and cut. This reinforcement is done now on the opposite side exactly the same way regardless of the presence of bone fractures. Upon completion the wound is again irrigated.

Next, the sutures bringing together the two halves of the sternum are placed. These are encircling double wires gauge 8 provided with long blunt needles that are placed in each intercostal space (Fig. 17.4). In smaller subjects the double wire may be substituted for single-strand wire gauge 8. At this point **before** tying these double

Fig. 17.4 Double-loop
wire gauge 8 placed
around the sternum lateral
to the reinforcing sutures

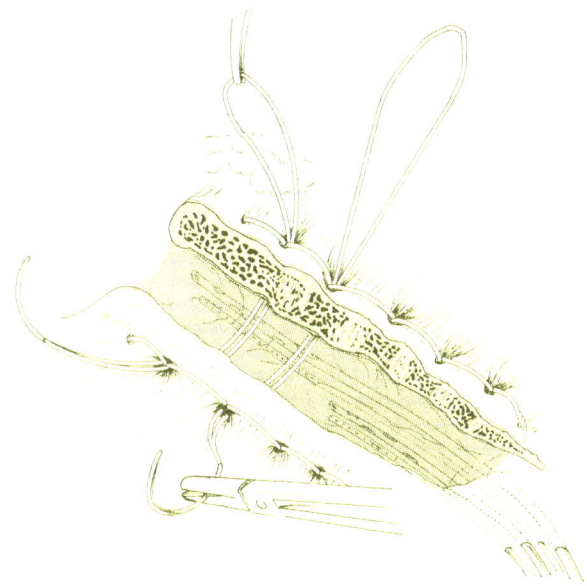

wires and irrigation-suction system are implanted in the retrosternal space
(Fig. 17.5). Two chest tubes size 24 are positioned in a staggered manner having the
tip of one at the manubrium level and the second tube is placed from the midportion
of the sternum down. Each tube is accompanied by a small parallel irrigating catheter placed in the same way. All four tubes exit the thoracic cavity through the
abdominal wall on the right side and are secured to the skin before the sternum is
closed. The wound is again irrigated.

Now the peristernal double wires are pulled together, twisted snugly, and cut.
The ends are buried in the deeper layers. A second superficial irrigating system is
now implanted over the sternum (Fig. 17.6). This superficial system is placed
exactly in the same staggered fashion as the deep system. This time however, all
four tubes are brought out through the upper abdominal wall on the left side. This
will help the nurses to know which of the suction/irrigating system is which. The
wound is once more irrigated. As the illustrations show, the peristernal double wires
exert pressure on the lateral reinforcing wires and not to the bone which is
protected.

To close the remaining subcutaneous and skin layer is done as a single layer with
a heavy-gauge monofilament suture. A Prolene number two with a large pointed
needle is preferred that embraces the skin and subcutaneous tissues in one single
layer in running fashion making sure that the skin is under no tension but approximated moderately snug keeping in mind that the irrigation system fluid to be implemented later will not leak to the outside through the suture line. Antibiotic ointment
is applied to the entire incision and the patient is transported to the intensive care
unit with all irrigation and suction systems functioning.

Fig. 17.5 A deep irrigating-suction system of catheters is positioned in a staggered manner behind the series of peristernal double wires (see text for details)

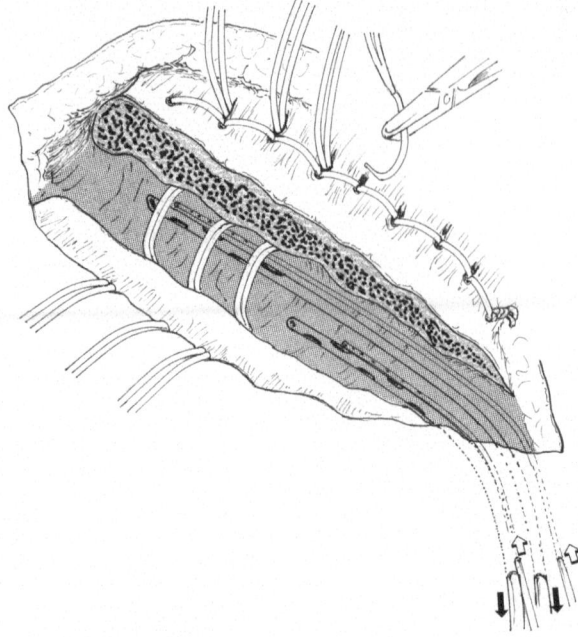

Fig. 17.6 After the sternum is approximated, another superficial staggered irrigation system is placed over the sternum. The single layer of skin/subcutaneous tissue is closed in a running fashion using size 2 Prolene suture (see text)

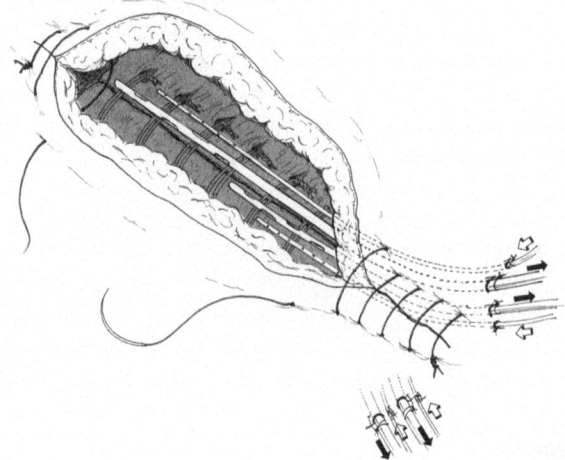

Stage 2: Postoperative Care

The patient has four catheters or tubes on each side of the upper abdomen. In order to impose a steady and reliable uniform amount of irrigation in each catheter, electrical infusion pumps are necessary (four of them) and not simple dripping by gravity. No "Y" connectors are permitted either. The rate of irrigation per catheter is set to 100 mL/h for the first 48 h. If at the end of that time the returning fluid has cleared with no debris or blood clots, then the irrigation rate may be decreased to 50 or 75/h. This is continued until the end of the first week. The only drawback at this stage is the large volume of fluid return; therefore the collecting containers must be replaced often. The patient is kept flat in bed and the head cannot be raised to more than 12°. A urinary catheter is kept in place throughout the first week. The patient is also kept on a low dose of prophylactic anticoagulant to prevent venous stasis and embolism. Usually Lovenox (low-weight heparin) at 40 mg/day subcutaneously is used and intermittent compressive pneumoboots are applied to both legs. The patient however may be moved side to side.

Once the 8 days post-op is reached the irrigations are discontinued and the irrigating catheters removed. The suction catheters stay in place. The patient is allowed out of bed only with assistance. He/she is not allowed to move the arms sideways or backwards, or over the head. Only anteriorly in front is permitted. The assistant nurse should stand at the foot of the bed and grasp the patient hands to help him/her to incorporate, to sit, and to move to a chair. Starting on the 8th day the chest suction tubes are advanced out 2 in. every day securing them with sutures looped under the skin stitch that was originally placed to secure the original tube. There is no need to place a new skin stitch every day. The antibiotic therapy continues without change or interruption.

Stage 3: Transfer to Regular Ward and Discharge

During the entire postoperative period the skin incision is left uncovered but cleansed twice/day with either Techni-Care or Hibiclens or its equivalent to prevent buildup of debris or dried-up crust that harbors bacteria. The skin suture remains in place for a total of 3 weeks. When all tubes are out, which takes about 1 week, the patient is discharged on antibiotic therapy for another 10 days and is asked to return for follow-up in 1 week to have the skin sutures removed. In our experience, the cure results were assured at 2 months post-op (Fig. 17.7).

One question may be this: How late after the original operation has this repair being done? Answer: It needs to be clarified. If the patient is referred from other facility and the dehiscence had occurred 1 year or more before but the incision has healed with or without implants of muscle flaps and there is no open wound and the patient has severe instability of the chest with almost continuous pain and discomfort, the repair can be done with the same success but the difference is that there was no infection and therefore all the patient needs is to have the repair operation. However being done so late has required more extensive mobilization for the following reasons: There were two patients who had had chest wall muscle flaps done by plastic surgeons to fill the sternal gap. However despite having skin grafts over this area, the disability of the patient persisted unchanged caused by instability of the chest, rendering the patients totally disable to work and having continuous chest wall pain. Implementing the repair as described above was difficult, tedious, and prolonged but the patients recovered well and returned to their occupation. There is,

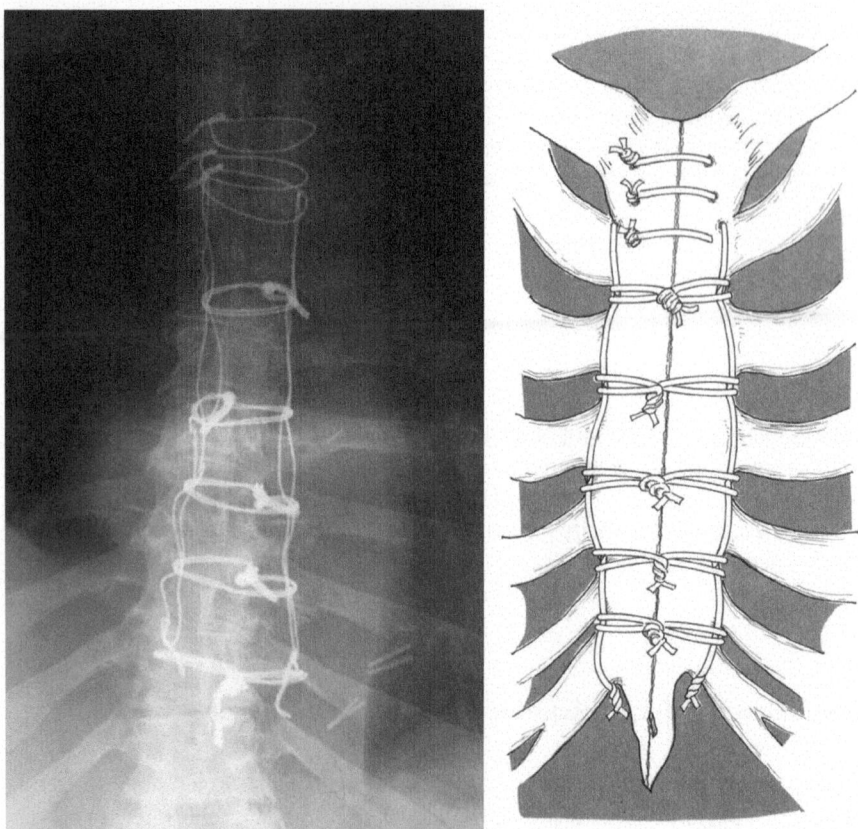

Fig. 17.7 Radiographic and drawing images showing how the closure must look to be effective at the end of the operation

therefore, no excuse for not attempting a total repair of the chest at any time, but "the sooner the better" (Fig. 17.8). Success in all cases treated can only be achieved when the protocol of care is strictly applied in all stages.

When the protocol described here is attempted but not done correctly the repair has to be redone as soon as the problem is seen. Some of our illustrations show the failures of improper repairs that cannot be blamed on the procedure itself but on the surgeon conducting it.

References

1. Ann Thorac Surg. 1993;55:459–63.
2. Ann Thorac Surg. 2004;78:912–7.
3. J Thorac Cardiovasc Surg. 2006;132:782–7.

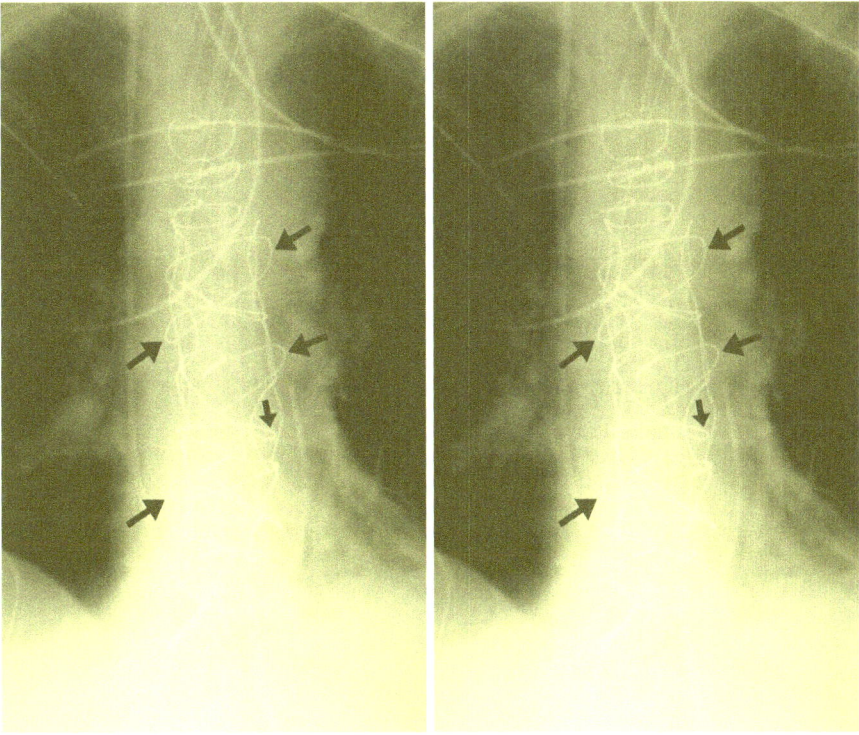

Fig. 17.8 Example of incorrect repair. The reinforcing wire does not reach the manubrium. The suture is loose and the peristernal wires at several levels do not touch the lateral reinforcing sutures. This repair failed a few days later and was redone with good results healing completely

Chapter 18
Prevention of Postoperative Sternal Dehiscence in Obese Patients

Obesity is still a serious problem in our American population. The reports of results of coronary bypass operations and in general of all types of cardiac operations in the adult population during the 80s and 90s had reported an average of 40% incidence of obesity. At present in years 2014–2015 the incidence of obesity has been reported at an increase of 65%.

This condition poses a significant challenge to the operating surgeon, because of not only higher risk of infection, respiratory complications, and drug dosage of medication, but also the precautions and measures that need to be taken to prevent dehiscence of the operative incision, more so if we consider the morbidity and mortality of a sternal dehiscence. One of the major problems frequently encountered is assessing to detect sternal instability to make the diagnosis in the early postoperative period. Even examining the patient on a daily basis, simple palpation of the sternal area is completely ineffective due to the extreme depth of the subcutaneous layer. When dehiscence is suspected a simple chest X-ray exam is useless and not contributory in clarifying the issue. The only radiologic studies of value are an overpenetrated X-ray of the dorsal spine or a CT scan of the chest. Those are the only two studies that will show whether displacement of the wire sutures has occurred or whether the sternal halves have separated.

There are some signs that may give the alarm to the surgeon that sternal dehiscence is developing. Among them is a constant pain in the operative area after 3 days when the patient starts activity. Routinely after this type of surgery the postoperative pain is more severe right after surgery but gradually it becomes more of a soreness after 2 or 3 days. But if the patients continues to complain of severe pain after that time, attention should be paid to the possibility of sternal dehiscence. The patient may report the feeling of a grinding sensation in the chest. Very rarely the patient may show some serous drainage from the incision but waiting for that sign to appear cannot be relied on.

In general as soon as the surgeon strongly suspects that sternum may be becoming unstable, the above-mentioned studies should be obtained and if some of those radiological signs are seen, or even if only the clinical impression seems to be very

© Springer International Publishing AG, part of Springer Nature 2018
J. E. Molina, *Cardiothoracic Surgical Procedures and Techniques*,
https://doi.org/10.1007/978-3-319-75892-3_18

suggestive, he/she should take the patient back to surgery for a revision of the entire incision. Most of the time the findings are found positive for dehiscence. Consequently, the sternum needs to be rewired but this time implementing the repair that is here recommended in order to prevent further deterioration and fracture of the bone at various levels. The more this approach is delayed the worse the results of repairing the incision and the risk for infection also increases proportionally.

Based on all this knowledge that we have dealing with this complication, the strong recommendation to any surgeon dealing with obese patients is to implement routinely a secure prophylactic reinforced closure as was described in the previous chapter. Exactly all the operative technical steps described in the previous chapter must be implemented.

At the time of the first operation, in our experience, any patient with a body mass index (BMI) of 30 or higher must undergo the lateral reinforcement of the sternum as described in the previous chapter, followed by the double-wire stitches used in every intercostal space to approximate the two halves of the sternum. It is of crucial importance that the reinforcing wires must be placed correctly as shown in a postoperative X-ray study (Fig. 18.1). The figures depicted in this chapter show a comparison between a wrongly performed reinforcement and one correctly done. In the first instance, the wrong repair had to be redone again. While placing the lateral reinforcing wire suture, it is somewhat hard to manipulate a wire gauge 8 because of its stiffness, but nevertheless it should be properly placed snugly.

Some technical points should be mentioned: When placing the lateral parallel reinforcing wire suture, careful dissection using the cautery should be used to clear each intercostal space flush to the sternum because when the circumferential peristernal double wires are placed, these stitches must pass exactly lateral to the parallel line of the reinforcing wire. In this manner the pressure of the encircling wire stitch is pulling wire against wire and not wire against bone. This is the reason why in obese individuals, the plain wire alone, thick as it may be, placed around the sternum will gradually cut through the bone in a few days, which does not occur with the technique described here. If the sternum in obese patients is always reinforced correctly, the surgeon does not have to be concerned about this complication.

With the experience in our institution operating on obese patients when other three types of sternal closures were implemented, it was found that the so-called figure-of-eight stitches, or the use of cables, or the simple peristernal mode, resulted in an incidence of dehiscence ranging from 7 to 8%. The details of the recommended technique are illustrated in the adjunct illustrations.

References

1. Ann Thorac Surg. 2004;78:912–7.
2. Ann Thorac Surg. 2001;71:521–31.
3. JAMA. 2001;286:1195–200.

Fig. 18.1 Detailed depiction of the prophylactic reinforced repair showing the double-loop wire running around the sternum lateral to the parallel reinforcing suture. Therefore the double wire exerts pressure on the wire and not on the bone

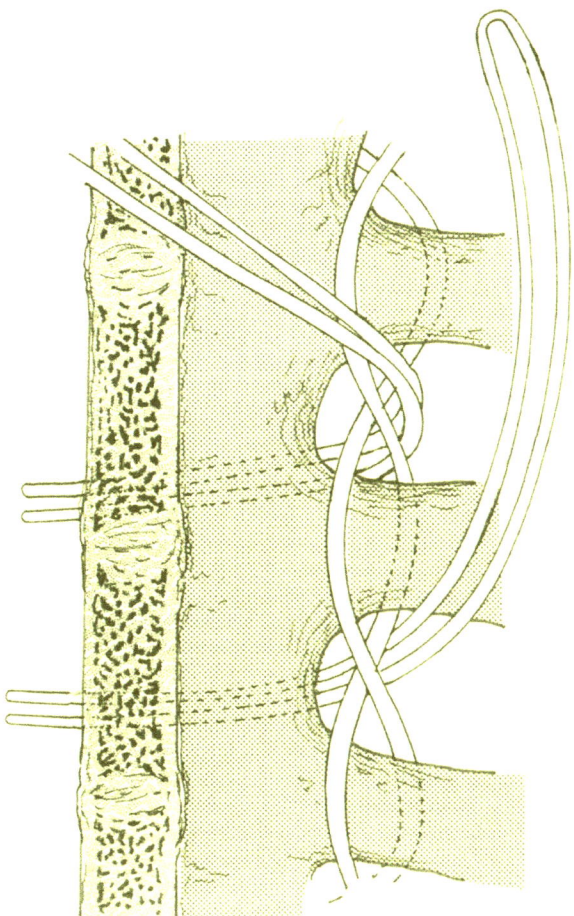

Part IV
Cardiology and Electrophysiology Advances

Chapter 19
Endocardial Pacemaker/Defibrillator Lead Implant Not Available to Cardiologists

When the standard intravenous route cannot be used for implanting pacemaker or defibrillator leads for various reasons, there are still surgical options which are not available to the electrophysiologist cardiologist. Most commonly the reason the intravenous route is not available is the total obstruction of the subclavian or innominate veins which has occurred due to repeated implants of leads throughout long periods of time, or due to placement of chronic central venous catheters for parenteral nutrition or for drug or antibiotic therapy. Presence of chronic dialysis catheters is another cause in patients with renal failure. The preferred route used by the cardiologist is the insertion of the lead in the left subclavian vein. In the case of defibrillator leads the reason attends also to have the pulse generator implanted on the left side of the upper chest to provide for an acceptable vector of the electrical current that travels from the pulse generator to the distal coils of the lead to defibrillate the heart. If the left-sided veins are occluded, the leads are then implanted via the right side. This change of routes, however, is often done more than once and the final result is that all venous access of the upper chest veins becomes unusable (Fig. 19.1). Therefore the surgeon is consulted to have an epicardial system of leads implanted. Such approach implies the performance of a thoracotomy, usually on the left side of the chest.

It is well known that the intravenous type of electrodes have better performance and durability than the epicardial type of leads. Therefore, if at all possible an endocardial lead is more desirable in the atrial and ventricular location.

The alternatives that can be offered by the cardiac surgeons to overcome the limitations that the cardiologist encounters are the transthoracic transatrial route and the internal jugular technique which are explained in the next section.

© Springer International Publishing AG, part of Springer Nature 2018   95
J. E. Molina, *Cardiothoracic Surgical Procedures and Techniques*,
https://doi.org/10.1007/978-3-319-75892-3_19

Fig. 19.1 Total obstruction of the subclavian, innominate veins and the superior vena cava. This is usually the result of multiple implants of pacemaker leads via intravenous routes

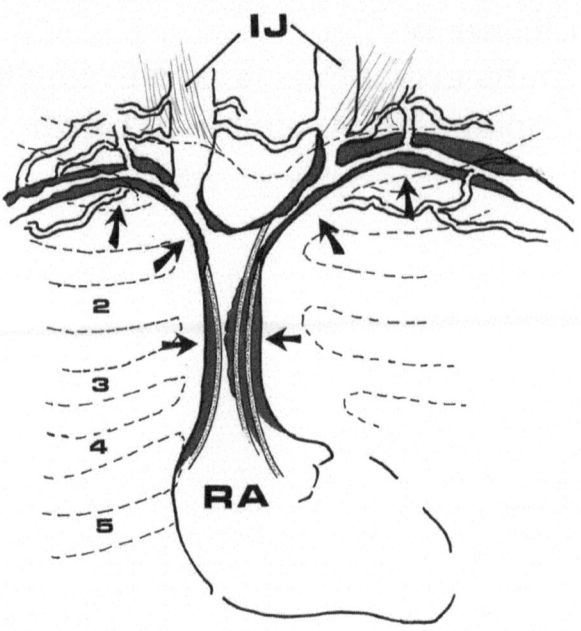

Chapter 20
Transthoracic Transatrial Approach

We call this method that has been developed the transthoracic transatrial approach (TTTA). Although the thoracic cavity is entered, it is very limited intervention that can be done without violating the pleural cavity in the majority of instances and also less painful postoperatively. The operation is conducted under general anesthesia and is described in detail in the following illustrations (Fig. 20.1).

With the patient in flat decubitus position fully anesthetized, the incision for this operation is made on the right side of the chest over the fifth rib extending it from the border of the sternum laterally for about 2 in. (Fig. 20.2). Later on, if needed, it can be extended. The subcutaneous tissue is entered, and the fibers of the pectoralis muscle are divided until the fifth rib cartilage is reached. The periosteum is stripped off the rib and the cartilage until this bone segment is totally free all around. The cartilage with the anterior portion of the rib is removed (Fig. 20.3). By careful blunt dissection detaching the mediastinal retrosternal tissue advancing medially without entering the pleura the pericardial membrane is identified. The internal thoracic vessels (mammary) are ligated at both ends and divided to provide the required space. Since many of the patients have had previous cardiac surgery the pericardium may not be intact. Otherwise a vertical incision is made in the pericardium and retaining sutures are placed in the free edges to provide for adequate exposure (Fig. 20.4). The right atrial wall is clearly exposed. A small purse-string suture with fine monofilament suture Prolene 4-0 is placed in its surface and a small tourniquet is applied to prevent bleeding (TTTA). The atrium is punctured in the center of the purse-string suture and, using the dilator provided with the kit, the pacemaker or defibrillator lead is inserted using the same type of dilator utilized for subclavian implants (Fig. 20.5). Under fluoroscopy monitoring the lead is positioned and anchored in the desired area of the atrium or apex of the right ventricle. The purse-string suture is tied. The free ends of the suture are also tied around the lead itself. If atrial and ventricular leads are required, then two purse-string sutures are placed and handled the same way (Fig. 1.3—TTTA). From here, the leads are tunneled to the site where the pulse generator is implanted. This could be on the right or left chest. If the pulse generator is located in the left upper chest, a tunnel is created behind the sternum

© Springer International Publishing AG, part of Springer Nature 2018   97
J. E. Molina, *Cardiothoracic Surgical Procedures and Techniques*,
https://doi.org/10.1007/978-3-319-75892-3_20

Fig. 20.1 The only route available is what we call the transthoracic transatrial approach (TTTA). Incision is made over the right fifth rib and cartilage

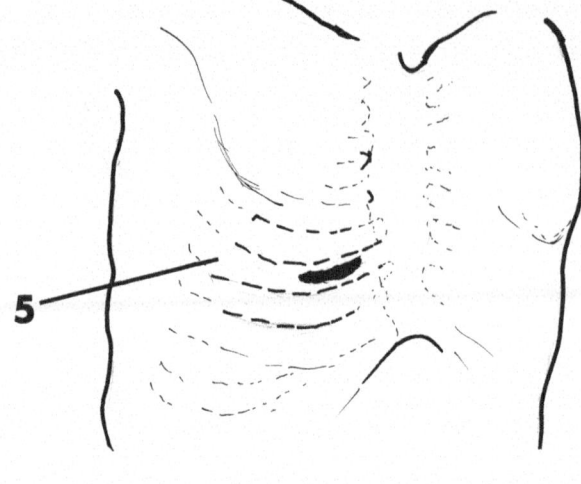

Fig. 20.2 The incision is carried over the fifth rib anteriorly toward the sternum

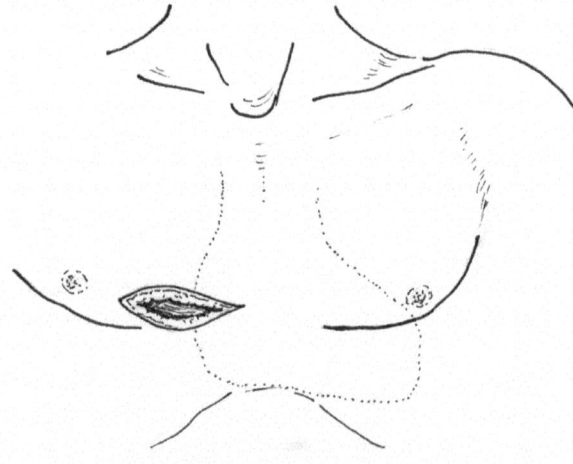

Fig. 20.3 The fifth rib and cartilage are exposed and removed for a short distance

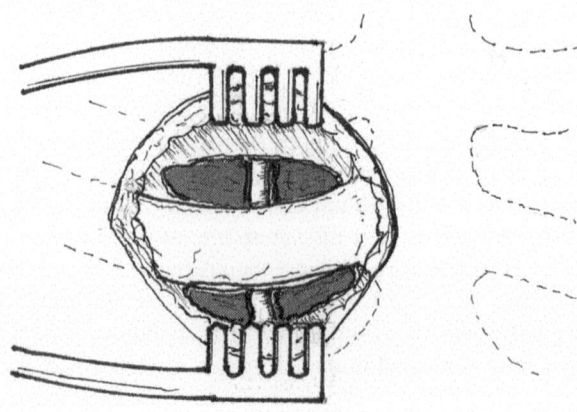

Fig. 20.4 Without entering the pleura the dissection progresses medially until the pericardium is reached and incised vertically exposing the right atrium. A purse-string suture is placed on the right atrial wall with 4-0 Prolene and the atrium is punctured

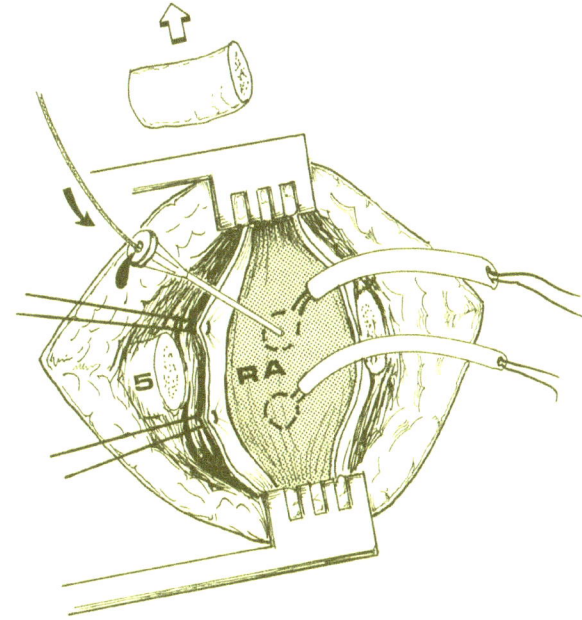

Fig. 20.5 The pacemaker or defibrillator lead or both are inserted using the usual equipment and the leads implanted. . Under fluoroscopic control the leads are positioned in the desired location and tested

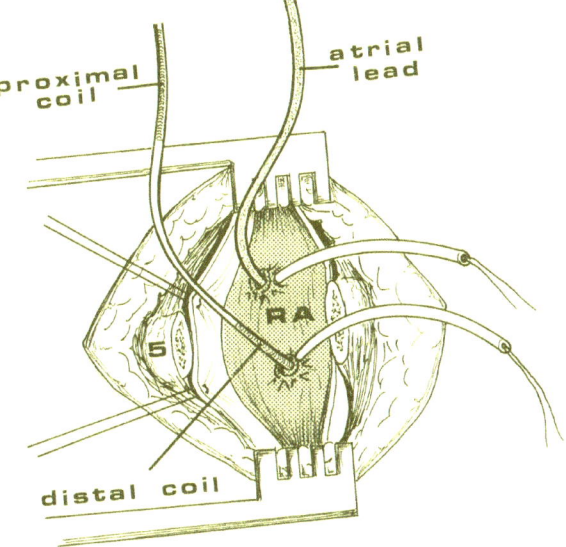

Fig. 20.6 This is an example showing the implanted defibrillator lead via TTTA approach, which is tunneled retrosternally to the level of the second left intercostal space and further tunneled to the site of the pulse generator implanted in the retropectoral space

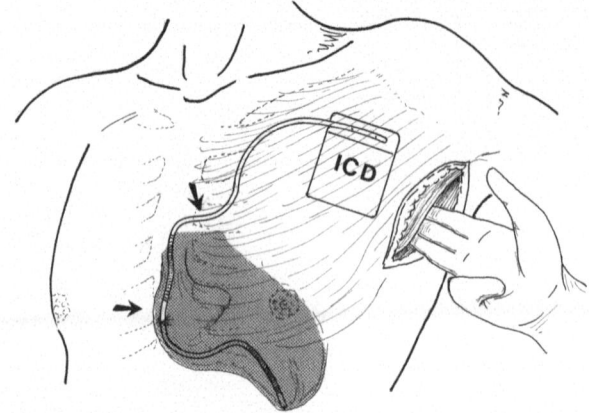

and not in the subcutaneous tissue. From that plane the second left intercostal space is reached. A small incision is made at that level to expose the tip of the pacer tunnel which is extracted bringing the connecting end of the lead with it. From that incision the lead is now directed to the site of the battery can. If the pulse generator is located on the right side, the lead is easily tunneled using the same instrument advanced under the pectoralis major muscle to that location. The chest incision is closed in the routine manner. If the pleural cavity was entered by accident a small chest catheter is implanted to allow for re-expansion of the lung (Fig. 20.6).

This described technique is direct, done under direct vision under highly sterile condition in a surgical suite. It should be preferred over some esoteric approaches described in the past like inserting pacing leads in the femoral vein and advanced via the inferior vena cava to reach the right-sided cardiac chambers. This approach should never be used for the obvious complications that carry such as thrombosis of the femoral vein with serious effects on the lower extremity causing chronic edema, obliteration of iliac vein, fibrosis, and stenosis of the inferior vena cava. It implies implant of pacer pulse generator in the abdominal wall and risks infections in the groin area and other complications such as break of the lead being subjected to continuous physical mobility of the entire system.

Chapter 21
Internal Jugular Approach

This surgical approach to implant pacemaker or defibrillator leads is only applicable if the innominate veins and the superior vena cava are still patent and the obstruction is limited to the subclavian veins (Fig. 21.1). This technique has been implemented also in children in whom the subclavian veins are electively not used due to their small caliber. It has always been recommended to obtain a duplex ultrasound exam or a CT angiogram scan in children being considered for intravenous pacemaker implants, because the minimal diameter of the subclavian vein must be 5 mm or greater to be able to accept a single intravenous pacemaker lead of 2 mm in diameter. This condition is not present until the child is 6 years of age or older. Therefore no subclavian implants of pacemaker single lead should be done in children younger than 6 years of age lest permanent obstruction of the subclavian vein will invariably occur.

If the internal jugular vein approach is selected for adults or for children, the operation is done by a cardiac surgeon following the steps that are described here and shown in the accompanied illustrations.

The fully anesthetized patient is positioned in decubitus and either the right or the left neck is exposed. A small transverse incision is made in the supraclavicular area lateral to the border of the sternocleidomastoid muscle (Fig. 21.2). Simultaneously, the area where the pacer pulse generator will be implanted should be prepped and draped. The platysma muscle is divided and the sternocleidomastoid muscle retracted medially. The soft tissues are entered and dissected until the anterior surface of the internal jugular vein is exposed. The **internal jugular vein does not have to be dissected around and isolated, nor tied off.** This is an error that risks to injure the phrenic nerve and compromises the venous return circulation from the head (Fig. 21.3).

A small purse-string suture is placed on the vein surface with a fine monofilament suture (Prolene 4-0) with a small tourniquet to prevent any bleeding. Using the standard kit for implanting pacemaker leads, the vein is punctured (Fig. 21.4). Using the dilator with the guide wire this latter is advanced for a short distance into the vein. This is followed by insertion of the pacemaker or defibrillator lead whichever

© Springer International Publishing AG, part of Springer Nature 2018   101
J. E. Molina, *Cardiothoracic Surgical Procedures and Techniques*,
https://doi.org/10.1007/978-3-319-75892-3_21

Fig. 21.1 When the subclavian veins are obstructed but the innominate and superior vena cava are patent, or the patient is a child older than 6 years, the internal jugular approach could be used

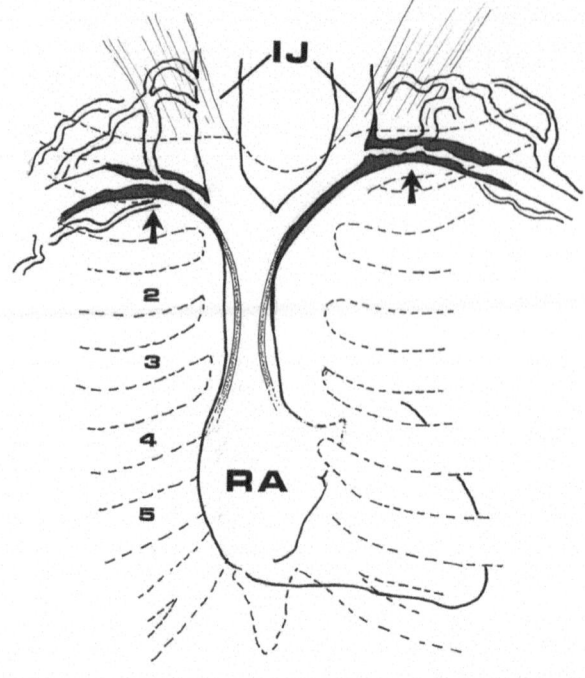

Fig. 21.2 A transverse incision is made in the supraclavicular area and simultaneously an incision is made in the lateral border of the pectoralis major muscle to enter the retropectoral space where the pulse generator will be implanted

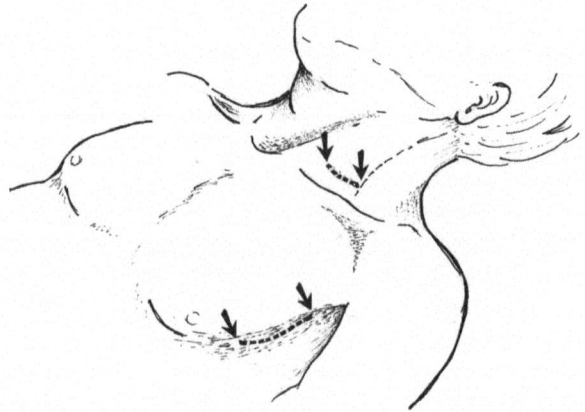

the case may be and under fluoroscopic control the lead is advanced into the innominate vein and superior vena cava until it reaches the cardiac chambers where the lead is positioned and anchored in the selected cardiac chamber (Fig. 21.5).

Now the purse-string suture in the jugular vein is tied snug to prevent bleeding and the free ends of the suture are tied to the lead itself and cut. Another suture with the same material but this time in the soft surrounding tissues is tied around the pacer lead itself to prevent dislodgement (Fig. 21.6) or migration.

Fig. 21.3 The internal jugular vein is exposed and without dissecting it all the way around and without tying it off, a small purse-string suture with fine material is placed with a tourniquet. The vein is punctured in the center

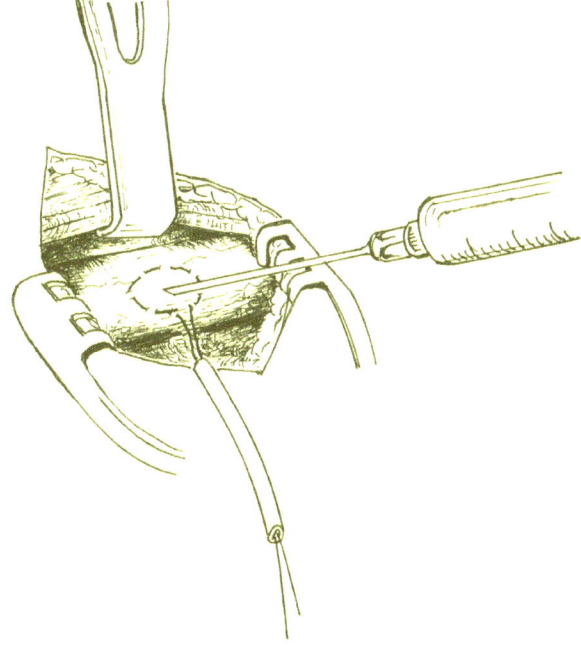

Fig. 21.4 Using the standard kit for inserting the guide wire, this is advanced in the internal jugular vein and superior vena cava

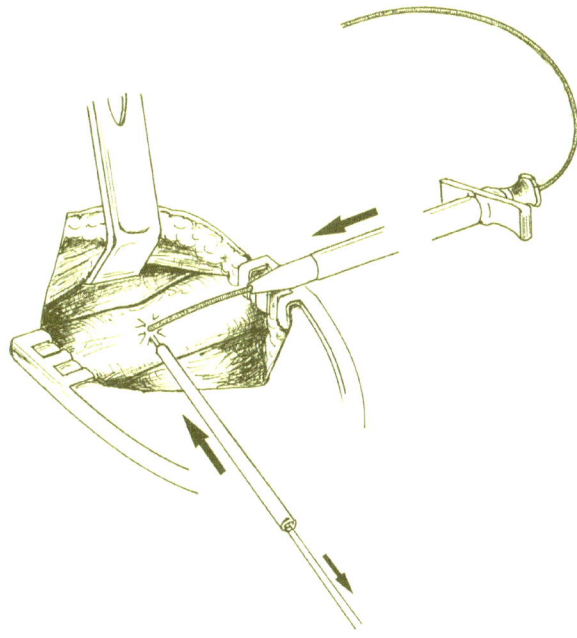

Fig. 21.5 The pacemaker or defibrillator lead is now inserted using the kit dilator

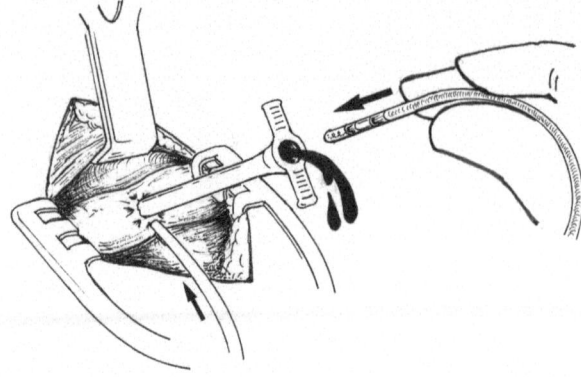

Fig. 21.6 Once the lead is anchored in the proper cardiac chamber using fluoroscopy, the lead is secured as shown (see the text)

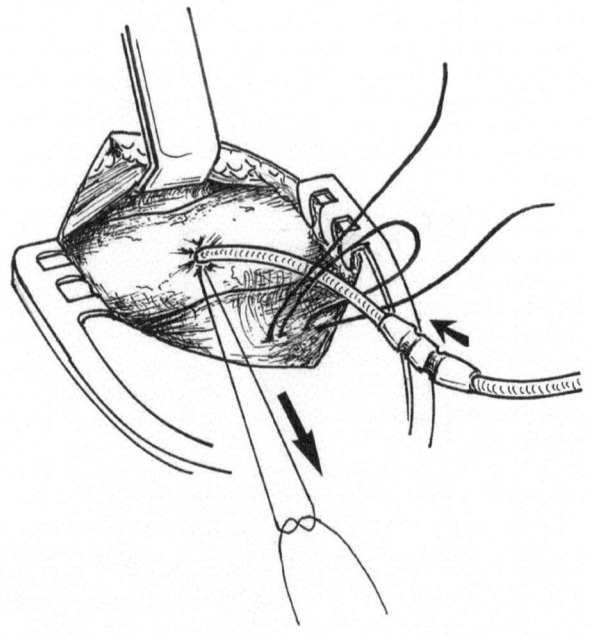

The next steps are aimed to connect the pacer/defibrillator lead to the pulse generator. These steps are very important depending on whether the patient is a child or an adult.

In an adult receiving only a pacemaker unit, the site where the pocket contains the pulse generator is created in the upper chest just below the clavicle. A transverse incision is made about 1–2 in. below this bone. A proper size space is created in the subcutaneous layer above and below the level of the skin incision large enough to receive the pulse generator. With blunt dissection using a hemostatic forceps a tunnel is made from the subclavicular pocket to the neck. **Always under the clavicle** (Fig. 21.7): This should be made as far lateral as possible in order to prevent any

Fig. 21.7 The lead now must be passed under the clavicle (never over) by creating a tunnel with a hemostatic clamp under the clavicle as far lateral as possible to avoid damage to the vessels and nerves

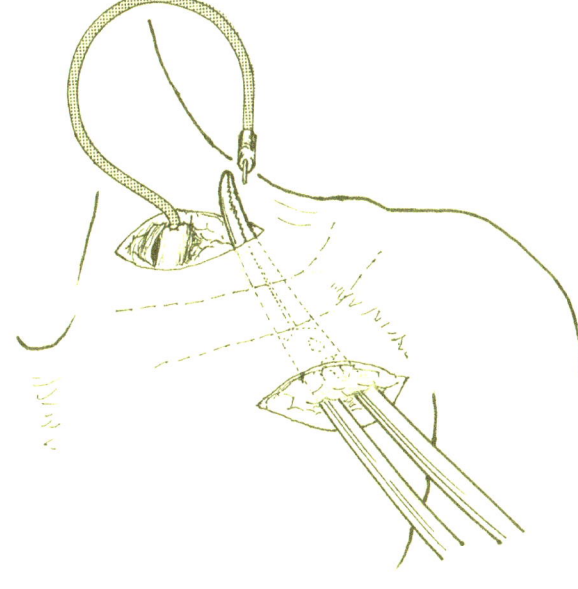

Fig. 21.8 If the pulse generator is planned to be implanted in the retropectoral space, this is created between the pectoralis major and minor muscles

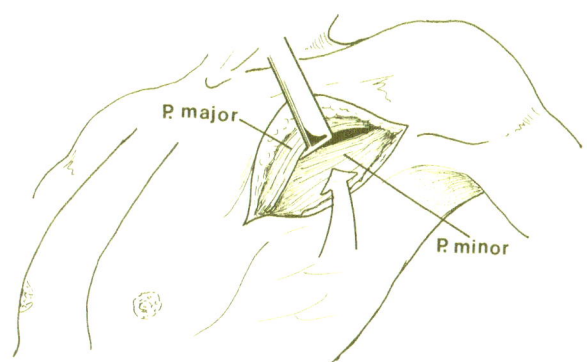

damage to the subclavian vessels that run underneath. Using a small catheter or drain tube (small chest tube usually suffices), the pacemaker/defibrillator lead can be placed inside it, to allow easy passage to reach the pocket. The lead is connected to the can and the incision is closed in the standard manner. In an adult receiving a defibrillator unit which is larger and heavier than a pacemaker, and also if the patient is an older child or a slender parson, the unit must be implanted in a retropectoral position to prevent erosion through the skin. Therefore a lateral incision is made along the lateral external border of the pectoralis major muscle. After entering the subcutaneous tissue (Fig. 21.8), the pectoralis major muscle is retracted medially and the dissection is continued over the pectoralis minor muscle. Therefore the space to be used to implant the pulse generator is between the pectoralis major and the pectoralis minor muscles. This is a large space able to accommodate the pulse generator which should be positioned as medial as possible toward the sternum. Now the lead is passed into this space and connected to the can. Once the pulse generator is in its final position the pocket must be closed laterally approximating the posterior aspect of the pectoralis major muscle to the anterior surface of the pectoralis minor. Four or five interrupted stitches of **nonabsorbable** suture material should be used to prevent migration of the unit. Absorbable material is not recommended because once the patient starts moving the arm, particularly in children, the pocket may work its way to the side after the suture material is dissolved, which could occur as early as 2 weeks. One of the most important points while making this operation is that the **pacemaker/defibrillator lead should not be passed over the clavicle. Always it must be passed under the clavicle**, be this adult or child, because if positioned over the clavicle the lead will erode through the skin sooner or later triggering a major disaster because if that happens the entire system will have to be removed.

The other important issue that the cardiologist must keep in mind is that if the pulse generator is placed behind the pectoralis major muscle, every time the pulse generator must be replaced—as the battery wears out—and the surgeon must be the person to undertake the replacement as well. However in the adult, when the pulse generator is superficial, in the subcutaneous tissue, the cardiologist may be able to do the replacement as long as the proper surgical techniques are followed under strict aseptic precautions that are observed to prevent infection which will be a serious event if it occurs.

References

1. J Interven Cardiac Electrophysiol. 2004;11;149–154.
2. Ann Thorac Surg. 1995;59;689–94.
3. Cardiac pacing and defibrillation: principles and practice.
4. Lu F. 2008. People's Med Publ House; pp. 476–490.

Chapter 22
The Infracardiac Defibrillator Lead Implant for Defibrillation Therapy

The implant of cardiac defibrillators to prevent sudden death in patients at risk, particularly patients with heart failure and candidates for cardiac transplantation, is frequently indicated. The practice of placing patch electrodes directly on to the heart was replaced many years ago by the less risky and obviously less invasive implant of intravenous leads. Currently the defibrillator lead consists of two active coils that receive the electrical impulse from the pulse generator needed to restore the normal rhythm to the heart. One coil at the end of the lead is positioned in the right ventricular chamber and the second coil is positioned in the innominate vein or upper superior vena cava. The lead is implanted usually via the left subclavian vein and positioned in the right ventricle anchoring the tip in the apex of the ventricle and the total length of the distal active coil is laid along the inferior wall of the right ventricular chamber.

Despite the capacity to program the pulse generator to the optimal electrical output to accomplish defibrillation of the heart, sometimes, even augmenting the potency of the shock the system fails or is only barely effective when the unit actually reaches the maximum energy that can deliver. In that situation the thought was that more leads were needed to create a wider area for the electrical current to surround the heart and hopefully be more effective. This attitude led to the practice of implanting leads in the subcutaneous tissue of the chest wall, some of them single and some with multiple arrays. However those leads cannot be implanted under local anesthesia and the procedure often becomes awkward as well.

Since the idea is to achieve an adequate position of the electrode coils to establish an electrical axis in which the electrical current crosses, as much as possible of the entire cardiac organ, but specifically the right and left ventricles, a new technique to accommodate this arrangement was designed in our institution that involves the placement of an infracardiac lead comprising both ventricles to accomplish this setting. What follows is a description of this method that does not require the use of

© Springer International Publishing AG, part of Springer Nature 2018
J. E. Molina, *Cardiothoracic Surgical Procedures and Techniques*,
https://doi.org/10.1007/978-3-319-75892-3_22

fluoroscopy monitoring. It is less invasive than a thoracotomy procedure and has shown to be quite effective in overcoming the limitations of the intravenous-alone arrangement. This approach has been utilized in patients who have had the intravenous system already implanted but had not been successful in defibrillating the heart adequately.

Implant of a Subcardiac Lead

The patient needs to be fully anesthetized and in decubitus position. An incision is made in the midline over the xiphoid process as described in the chapter on cardiac tamponade. The xiphoid process is removed and by doing blunt dissection the soft tissues in the pre-peritoneal space are retracted downwards until the pericardium is identified (Fig. 22.1). A transverse incision is made in the pericardium to gain adequate access to the infracardiac space.

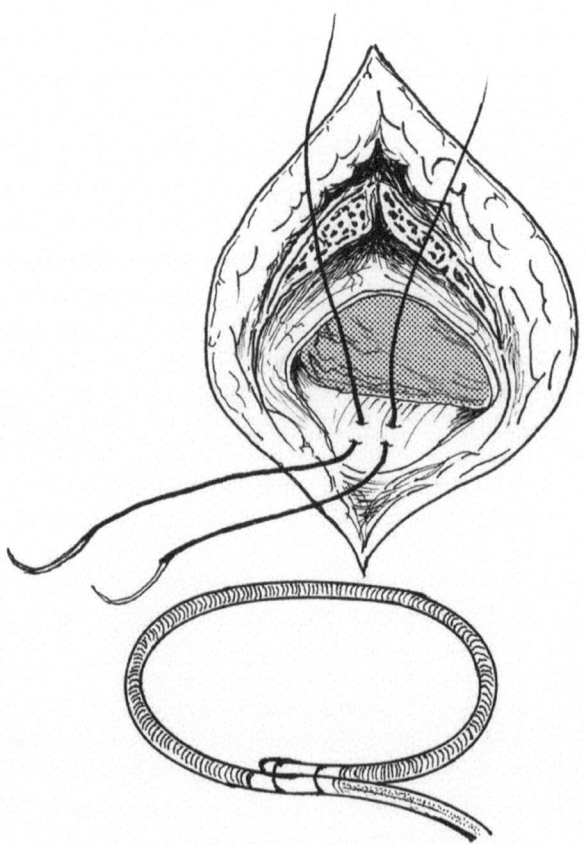

Fig. 22.1 A trans-xiphoid incision is made to expose the pericardium . This is incised transversally and two 2-0 stitches are placed on the diaphragmatic surface of the pericardium. The "halo" lead has already been constructed (see the description in the text)

Description of the Lead

At present, there is no specific defibrillator lead manufactured by any company designed for this use. Therefore a lead manufactured by Medtronic Inc. (Minneapolis, MN, USA) for subcutaneous use has been adapted for this new operation. The lead 6996-SQ is modified as follows: Before implant, the metal stylet inside the lead is extracted and measured in its entire length. Then, the portion of the stylet corresponding to the length of the defibrillation coil is cut with a wire cutter but is saved for the following step. The short piece already cut is now inserted in the lead and using the rest of the stylet this is also inserted behind in order to push the cut portion to reach the end of the lead. This must be precisely measured by checking the remaining intact portion of the stylet that has shoved the cut section inside the lead. The pusher stylet is removed. The portion of the lead containing the defibrillator coil is folded upon itself to form a halo (circle) which measures 7–8 cm in diameter. The halo is secured firmly now with a double tie of nonabsorbable suture (Fig. 22.1). Remember that the coil has now inside the short portion of stylet which makes the halo rigid and stable to maintain its round form. The rest of the lead remains pliable once the rest of the stylet (the pusher) is removed. The "halo" lead is now ready to be positioned in the pericardium under the heart.

Two stitches with nonabsorbable suture material (Ethibond 2–0) are placed on the diaphragmatic surface of the pericardium but not tied at this point. By gently lifting the right ventricle, the "halo" lead is now slid under the heart aimed to comprise the inferior wall of the left and right ventricles (Fig. 22.2). The sutures are now

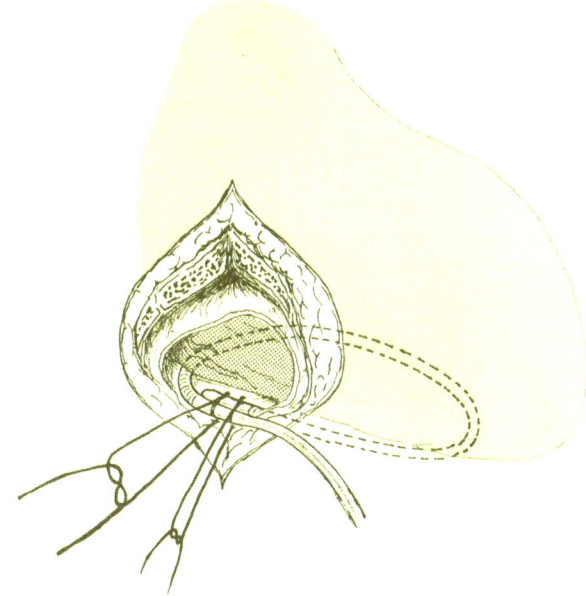

Fig. 22.2 The lead is slid under the heart and the sutures are tied to secure it in place

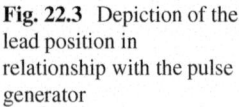
Fig. 22.3 Depiction of the
lead position in
relationship with the pulse
generator

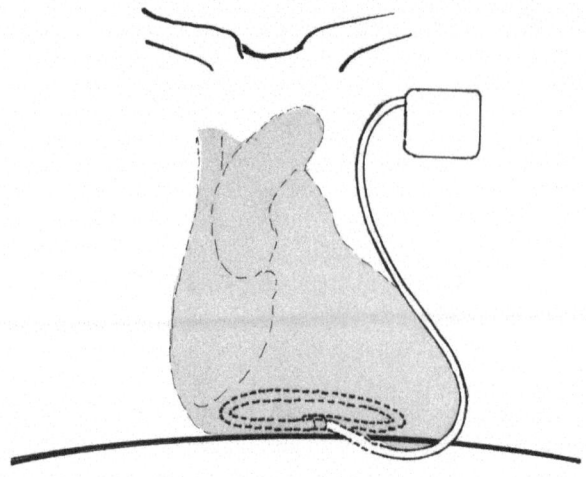

tied to secure the lead in place. From that point on, the rest of the lead is now tunneled in the subcutaneous tissue to reach the site of the pulse generator to which it is connected (Fig. 22.3).

This arrangement creates a straight electrical axis from the pulse generator to the lead comprising the entire heart, right and left ventricles. This design was initially tested in lambs and, after observing the reliability of its function, lack of deformity, or migration after prolonged period of observation, it was concluded that in such difficult and insolvable clinical cases, a clinical trial was indicated.

In 2004 the results of five such cases were reported. All of them had the intravenous system implanted, three of them with subcutaneous leads and two of them being back several times to attempt defibrillation with more powerful generators. A 78-year-old man also had had a subcutaneous patch implanted previously but after testing six configurations for defibrillation using 32 J all of them failed. Replacing the generator for one of higher output namely the Marquis DRICD model 7274 Medtronic called GemDR model 7271 all attempts failed and the patient had to be rescued with various external rescue shocks.

Implanting the "halo" lead, a single 24 J discharge defibrillated the patient on the first attempt and remained constant on subsequent tests.

Another patient, a 19-year-old woman, awaiting heart transplantation already with subcutaneous leads in addition to the intravenous system could not be defibrillated with up to 35 J. She was given the "halo" lead system and was effectively defibrillated at the first attempt with 25 J shock. Our new system therefore is obviously superior to the intravenous arrangements. In two of our patients, the electrophysiologists disconnected the intravenous leads altogether keeping only the subcardiac unit active.

It is our contention based on the results of this new approach that this system should be probably implanted as a first choice over the intravenous lead system. In addition the operative technique does not require the use of fluoroscopy but only

Fig. 22.4 X-ray study in a patient with previous transvenous defibrillator leads in the right ventricle and the "halo" lead under both ventricles. The pulse generator can be seen in the right upper corner

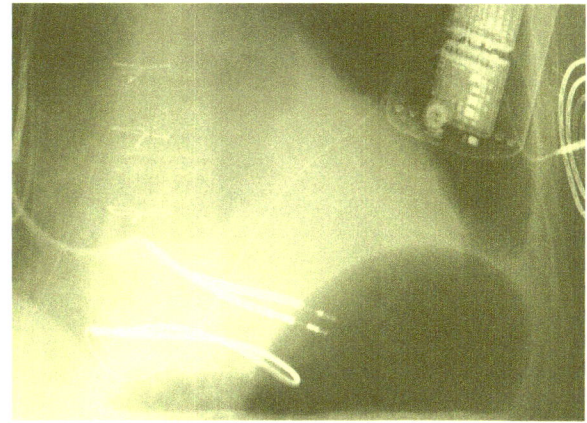

intraoperative testing after the implant. The only complementary intravenous lead is for sensing to monitor the cardiac rhythm to activate the generator when needed. Placing the subcardiac "halo" lead takes about 20 min and the entire operation approximately 1 h. The main advantage of this procedure is the incorporation of the left ventricle in the circuit which is not attained with the intravenous technique.

A radiographic view shows the position of the leads implanted in one case and also the straight electrical axis from the pulse generator to the infracardiac "halo" lead that makes the system so effective in its function (Fig. 22.4). The surgical intervention is well tolerated.

References

1. PACE. 2004;27:1500–1506.
2. J Interven Cardiac Electrophysiol. 2004;11:149–154.
3. Cardiac pacing and defibrillation: principles and practice. Lu F (editor). 228 People's Medical Publishing House; pp. 476–490.

Chapter 23
Standby for Cardiology when Chronic Pacemaker or Defibrillator Lead Removal Is Undertaken

Cardiac surgeons are often asked, by the electrophysiologist cardiologist, to assist as a backup team resource when old chronically implanted pacemaker or defibrillator leads are being removed via intravenously with the laser technique, if for any reason their procedure becomes seriously complicated.

The intravenously implanted leads gradually become firmly adherent to the endothelial surfaces of the cardiac chambers as well as to the vein walls. However some leads may be removed by manipulations and traction when the date of their implant has been relatively recent. Once the lead has been in place for years, it is firmly attached to the endovascular walls and its removal requires either a surgical approach or the use of a laser-guided system that can cut through the fibrous tissue surrounding the lead to release it.

The risks of tearing or rupturing the venous vascular channels or cardiac chamber walls particularly the atrium are very real, particularly the right atrial wall. Trusting their ability to accomplish this procedure under fluoroscopic control the cardiologist requests the surgical team to be available to rescue the patient if a catastrophe occurs.

However the manner in which this "coverage" is arranged is often inadequate, ineffective, or totally wrong. When the right atrial wall, superior vena cava, or innominate vein is torn, the patient goes immediately into shock in a matter of 2 or 3 min and if the hemorrhage cannot be controlled within minutes cardiac arrest follows and the patient may die right in the procedures room.

Having the surgeon on "standby" does not mean that when the intervention is being undertaken, the surgical team is somewhere in the hospital to be called when the complication happens. Being in the proximity of the operating room or in the hallway outside of the operating room is not sufficient. This is completely inadequate and useless because by the time the surgeon arrives, scrubs, dresses up, enters the surgical room, and undertakes the sternotomy to reach the site of the injury, long minutes have gone by and no less than 15 or 20 min have past. That is a critical time, without mentioning even longer time if the patient needs to be placed on cardiopulmonary bypass when the perfusion team is not ready. Many patients have died due

© Springer International Publishing AG, part of Springer Nature 2018   113
J. E. Molina, *Cardiothoracic Surgical Procedures and Techniques*,
https://doi.org/10.1007/978-3-319-75892-3_23

to the poor planning of this intervention, or have suffered brain damage if they survive.

Several considerations should be evaluated. First of all, the cardiology team should fully evaluate the indications for the lead removal. Is it necessary to contemplate removal of old chronically implanted lead with the risks involved? Are there other options like implanting an additional lead without removing the old one? Can an epicardial lead be implanted by the surgeon instead if the intravenous route cannot be used?

In the next chapter there are descriptions of other alternative methods to implant new leads that are available to the cardiac surgeon but not to the cardiologist. Therefore there should be a communication between the cardiologist and the surgeon in advance to decide about the best way to proceed. The cardiologist may not be aware about these other techniques to overcome the limitations of the currently intravenous routes that are the only ones available to him/her.

The patient must be fully aware and informed of potential complications including possibility of requiring a major operation and also of dying if things go wrong.

If the indication for removal is the only option available, then the intervention needs to be properly planned with the cooperation of the surgeon. When the request is made for a surgical standby, the only pertinent and safe way is as follows:

1. The proper surgical preparation of the patient must be implemented. After the patient is anesthetized (general anesthesia is always necessary) the chest must be shaved, prepped, and draped.
2. The surgeon or surgical team must be fully scrubbed and gowned ready to intervene standing on the opposite side of the cardiologist ahead of any manipulations.
3. Blood should be available in the room and the perfusion team must be ready to implement extracorporeal circulation if this becomes necessary.
4. The proper surgical instruments must be ready on the nurse instrument table including a sternal saw.
5. If the lead removal is successful, the patient needs to be observed nevertheless for several minutes to assure that no complication has occurred before the patient is taken back to the recovery room.

In the experience in our institution implementing the above plan of prevention, in four cases where this complication occurred, the time that took to control the hemorrhage was 4–6 min. In no instance the use of cardiopulmonary bypass was necessary and all the patients survived without neurologic damage.

In our opinion, following the above steps is the only acceptable method of preventing fatalities that may be associated with removal of chronically fibrosed intravenous pacer or defibrillator leads, when using laser-guided intravenous technique implemented by the cardiologist.

Part V
Vascular Surgery Procedures and Techniques

Chapter 24
Subclavian Vein Thrombosis
Paget-Schroetter Syndrome

This topic is of great importance because incorrect care of these patients is still happening today although the effective treatment with 100% success has been published several years ago. If not treated promptly the patients are left with significant permanent disability of several degrees.

Subclavian vein thrombosis is usually an acute event related to the recurrent compression of the vein by physical activity caused by professional work done with the arms seen in mechanics, construction workers, carriers or lifters of heavy objects or also by sports like tennis players, weight lifters, swimmers, baseball pitchers, and others. Therefore the syndrome is seen more often in young people from 15 to 45 years of age, but it may occur in older people involved in similar activities. The treatment must always be handled as an emergency.

The patients affected by this condition develop sudden pain and severe edema of the affected arm (Fig. 24.1) due to the obstruction of the arm venous return circulation. This is a condition that requires prompt diagnosis and always emergency type of care, because once the thrombosis sets in, the thrombotic process progresses distally very rapidly into the arm veins as well as centrally toward the innominate vein and occasionally is the source of pulmonary embolism (Fig. 24.2). The damage of the vein becomes severe in very short time. It evolves in fibrosis with severe or total obliteration with disappearance of its lumen. Therefore the treatment must be undertaken immediately.

The surgical procedure is described and illustrated here; however the complete treatment involves three stages namely (1) lysis of the clot followed by (2) the surgical operation to decompress the vein and reestablish its original caliber, and (3) anticoagulation for 8 weeks to prevent recurrence and permanent cure.

© Springer International Publishing AG, part of Springer Nature 2018   117
J. E. Molina, *Cardiothoracic Surgical Procedures and Techniques*,
https://doi.org/10.1007/978-3-319-75892-3_24

Fig. 24.1 Clinical presentation of a man with acute right subclavian vein thrombosis

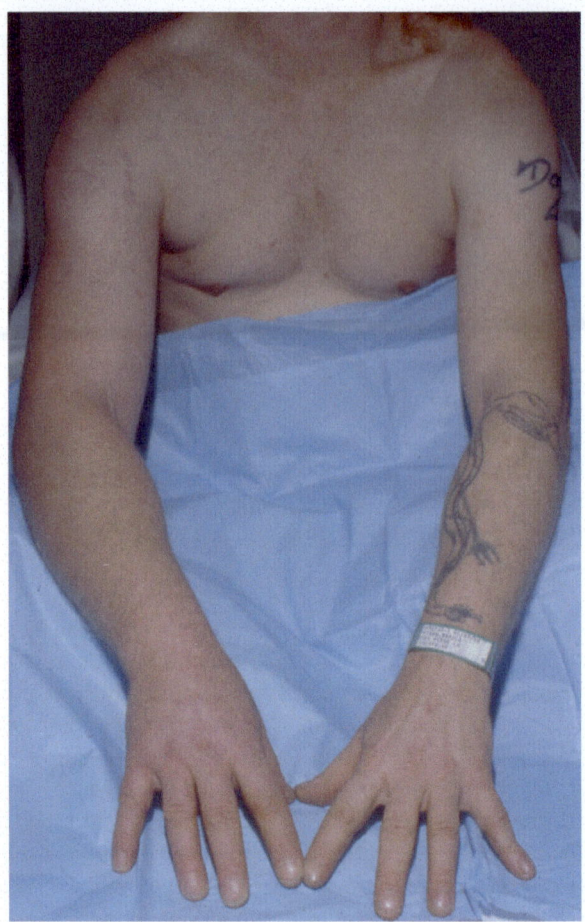

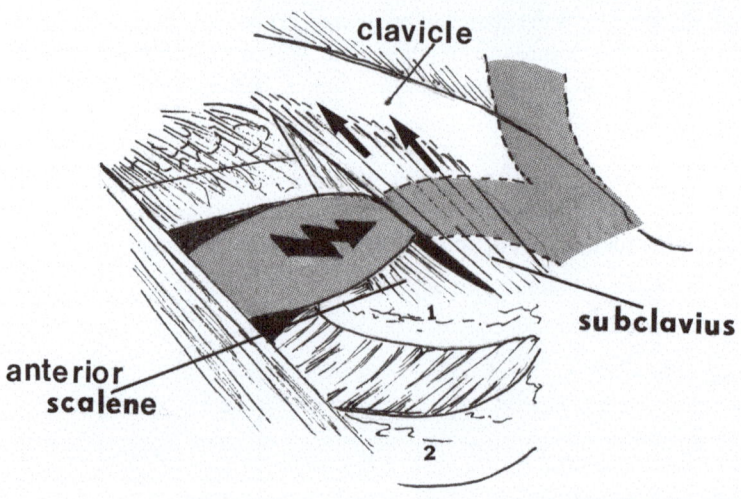

Fig. 24.2 The mechanism of sudden obstruction of the subclavian vein occurs when the subclavius muscle goes on tension against the anterior scalene muscle behind, and the first rib below

The Approach to Complete Treatment

Stage I

The patient must be hospitalized immediately and the diagnosis made by obtaining an ultrasound exam of the subclavian vein. Next, upon confirmation of the diagnosis the interventional radiologist must be contacted for a venogram study to show the extent of the thrombosis (Fig. 24.3) and, in the same session, an infusion catheter is positioned in the subclavian clot to begin a continuous infusion of a thrombolytic agent: tenecteplase (TNK), alteplase, or similar lytic agent chosen by the radiology team. The infusion must be implemented with an electrical pump for accuracy. The dose is adjusted to 0.05 mg/Kg/h. This averages to 0.25 mg/h. TNK has been found safe and affordable. A clot is usually dissolved in less than 24 h (Fig. 24.4). Once the vein is clean, the extent of the vein stenosis is assessed by repeated venography. Now the patient is ready for the stage II of treatment which entails the surgical

Fig. 24.3 A venogram is obtained and the interventional radiologist places an infusion catheter in the clot to implement thrombolytic therapy which is instituted immediately (see text)

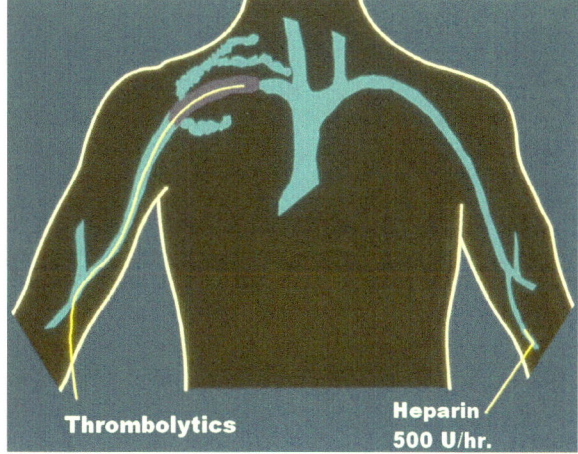

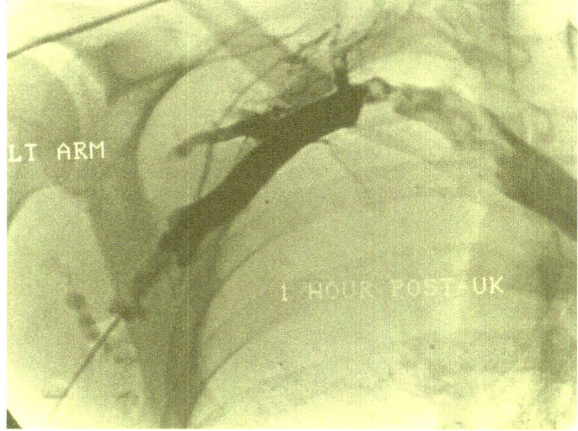

Fig. 24.4 After a short time, usually less than 24 h, the clot is lysed and the obstruction in the vein is clearly visualized

repair. NO STENTS SHOULD BE PLACED AT THIS STAGE. This has been an error committed in the past that does not solve the problem because the primary mechanism that led to the vein thrombosis is the mechanical extrinsic compression of the vein by the muscles and tendons of the thoracic outlet surrounding it. SURGICAL DECOMPRESSION MUST BE DONE FIRST. If a stent is placed at this stage, it will collapse as soon as the balloon of the catheter is deflated and also the vein is further damaged by this trauma; moreover, if the surgical decompression is undertaken at that point, it becomes a much more complex issue; thus the stent cannot be removed without inflicting severe injury to the vein which will be impossible to repair.

Stage II

The thrombolytic infusion is stopped and the patient is taken to the operating suite 3–4 h after, allowing sufficient time for the thrombolytic activity to wear off. If the patient cannot be operated when requested, then it should be maintained on a heparin infusion that is to be stopped 2 or 3 h before the time of surgery. The steps of the surgical procedure are illustrated in the following sequence: A transverse subclavicular incision is made (Fig. 24.5) about 2 in. below the clavicle. The fibers of the pectoralis major muscle are split in their direction and the adipose tissue beneath is removed. This approach exposes the area with the important structures to be identified (Fig. 24.6).

The subclavius muscle tendon is immediately found in front inserting on the first rib. It covers the medial portion of the subclavian vein (Fig. 24.7). Therefore the muscle is dissected off the vein, divided, detached, and lifted toward the back until its insertions are severed under the clavicle. The muscle is removed totally. This maneuver exposes the entire anterior surface of the subclavian vein and one can see the indentation made on the vein with some inflammatory tissue and fibrosis at the

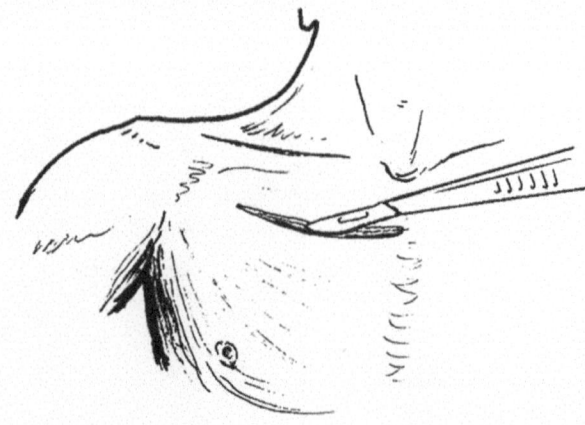

Fig. 24.5 A transverse incision is made about 2 in. below the clavicle on the affected side

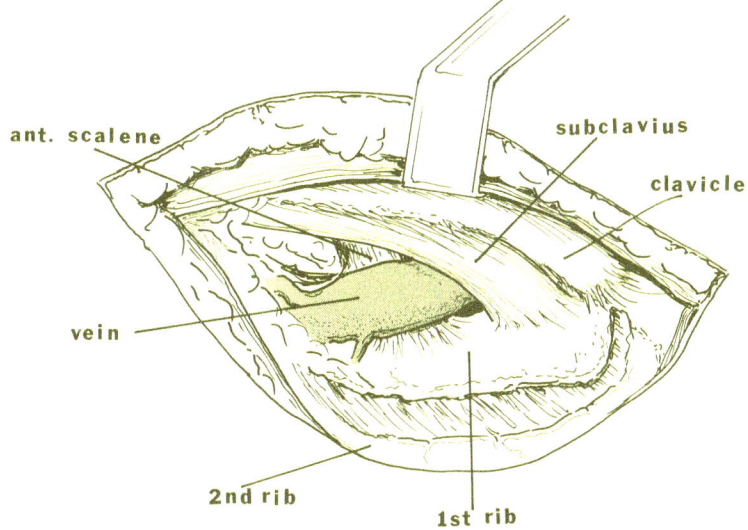

Fig. 24.6 After going through the skin, subcutaneous tissue layer, and splitting the fibers of the pectoralis major muscle, the important structures involved are shown

Fig. 24.7 The subclavius muscle is approached first at its point of insertion in the first rib

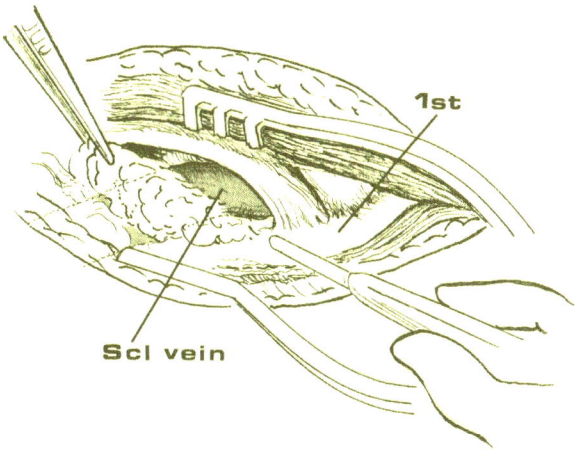

site of the constriction (Fig. 24.8). The vein is gently lifted up off the rib surface. The first rib is now approached for its removal.

An incision with the cautery is made along the inferior border of the first rib, and with a periosteal elevator the inferior surface of the rib is dissected without entering the pleura (Fig. 24.9). Once sufficient space is created under the rib, a digital exploration detaches the soft tissues off the extrapleural space (Fig. 24.10). This maneuver is very important in order to prevent a pneumothorax when the anterior scalene muscle tendon is divided. Now, retracting the vein superiorly to protect it, a

Fig. 24.8 The subclavius tendon is divided and the muscle reflected upwards resecting it completely from the inferior surface of the clavicle

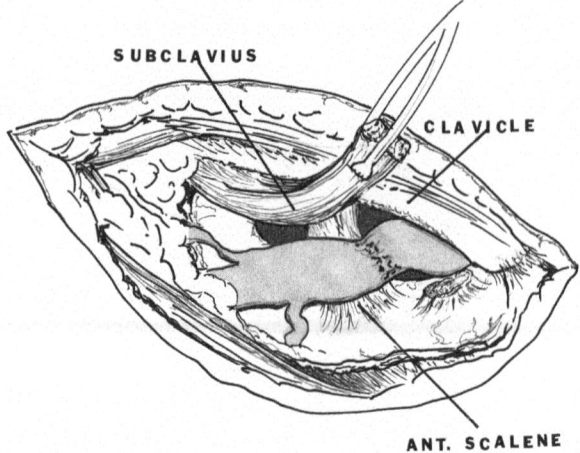

Fig. 24.9 The first rib must now be removed. Therefore a subperiosteal dissection is undertaken from the front to the back without entering the pleural space. *1st* first rib, *2nd* second rib, *Scal ant* anterior scalene muscle

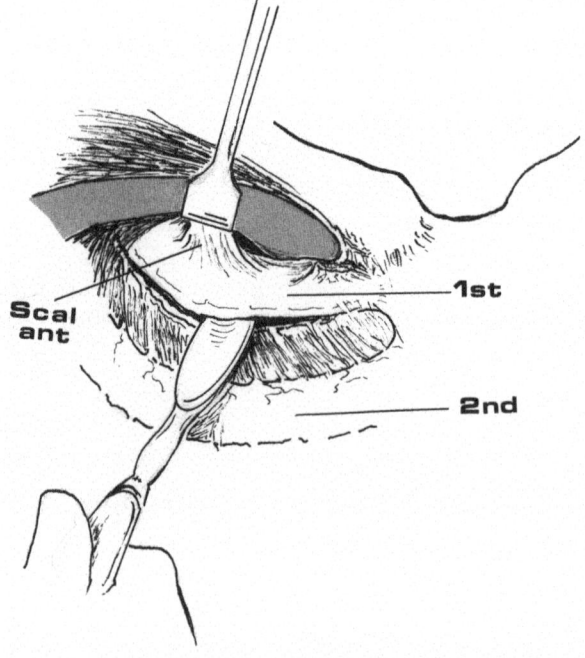

right-angled forceps is passed around the anterior scalene muscle tendon and divided (Fig. 24.11) detaching it totally off the rib. The first rib can now be divided, first anteriorly as close as possible to the sternum (Fig. 24.12) and also at the posterior end (Fig. 24.13). The patient is given a single dose of heparin (100 U/Kg) and the vein is clamped distally and proximally beyond the site of the obstructed segment (Fig. 24.14). The vein is opened crossing the obstructed segment, cleaned

Fig. 24.10 Digital maneuver completes freeing up the inferior surface of the rib. This maneuver is very important before attempting to divide the tendon of the anterior scalene muscle just behind the vein. This will prevent causing pneumothorax while trying to divide the anterior scalene muscle. That will happen if this sequence of steps is not followed. *Scl* subclavian vein, *Sub mus* subclavius muscle resected

Fig. 24.11 The anterior scalene muscle tendon is divided while retracting the subclavian vein superiorly. A right-angle forceps is passed around the tendon and cut

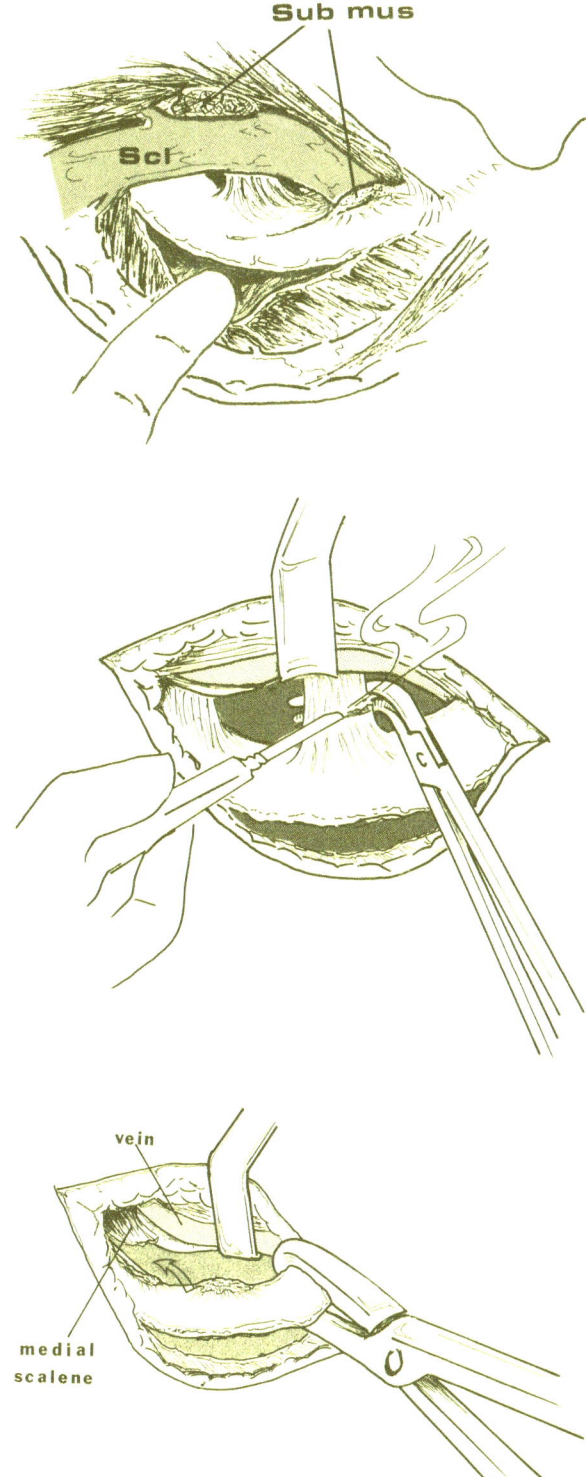

Fig. 24.12 Retracting the vein out of the way, the rib is divided anteriorly

Fig. 24.13 The posterior end of the rib is divided and the rib is removed

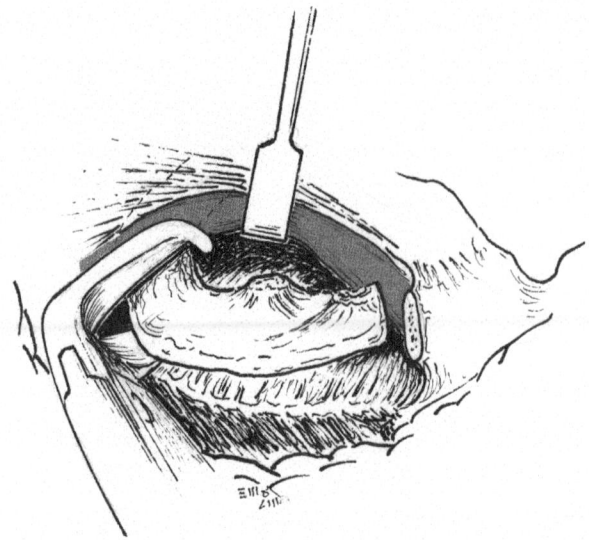

Fig. 24.14 Having the vein totally freed, particularly detaching it from the posterior aspect of the sternum medially, it can now be opened and repaired. Two vascular forceps are required: one is placed on the axillary vein and the other on the medial end of the subclavian

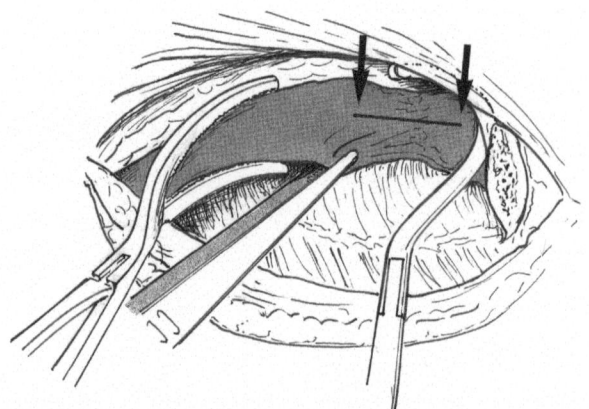

from residual thrombus, synechiae, and residual fibrous tissue (Fig. 24.15). A previously tailored piece of harvested saphenous vein from the thigh to provide larger diameter is brought into the field and laid over the venotomy. It is sutured in place as a patch and the clamps are released.

Stage III

This stage is as important as the previous two. Once the operation is terminated, a drain is positioned in the extrapleural space (usually a Jackson-Pratt type size 19) and the incision closed.

Fig. 24.15 Upon opening of the vein, old organized thrombus is removed as well as synechia is often found. The vein is cleaned and irrigated with heparinized saline. A segment of previously harvested saphenous vein is sutured over the stenotic area increasing its diameter to a normal size

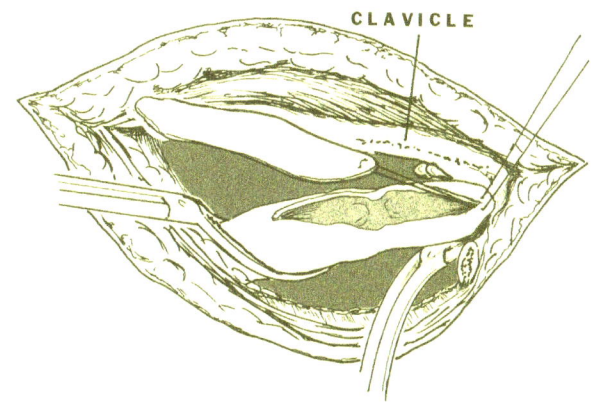

Fig. 24.16 Postoperative venogram shows the lpatent vein without any obstruction. In this case an intravascular stent was implanted by the radiologist because an area of residual obstruction was identified

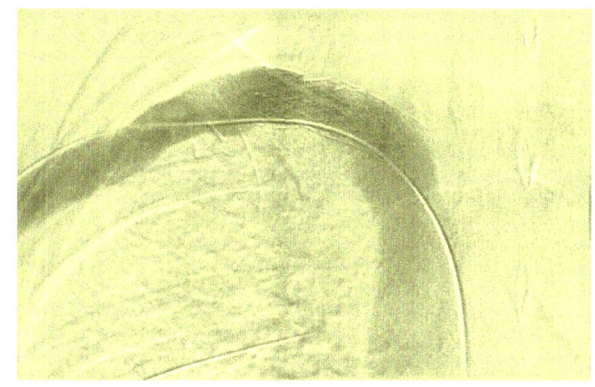

A postoperative venogram must be obtained within 24 h after surgery and the patency of the repair verified (Fig. 24.16). If any residual stenosis still persists, which is very common, the radiologist should proceed to dilate it and implant a stent which at this point is safe because the extrinsic compression to the vein has been eliminated and no risk exists of the stent collapsing (Fig. 24.16). The point should be stressed that balloon **dilation alone is not effective** because the stricture present is formed by fibrous tissue, and this will invariably restrict again within very few days. Placement of stent is the only proper intervention to undertake.

The patient needs to be anticoagulated for 6–8 weeks. Therefore the same evening of the operation day coumadin at a dose of 10 mg and plavix at 75 mg are administered until the proper level is reached. A range of 2–3 INR is sought to be maintained for the following 6–8 weeks. However because the optimal level of anticoagulation is not reached until about 48 h after surgery, enoxaparin 40 mg is administered subcutaneously twice a day until the proper INR is attained.

After the drain is removed and the patient discharged the follow-up is accomplished with ultrasound exam. At the end of 6–8 weeks all anticoagulants are discontinued and the patient resumes his/her normal activities.

The surgeon must be aware of the possibility that after opening the obstruction of the subclavian vein, he/she cannot reach adequate normal proximal subclavian vein to lay the vein patch appropriately and if the fibrous obstruction of the vein extends more medially under the sternum, then the surgical incision needs to be extended further into the sternum to reach the innominate vein. This technique is fully described in the next Chap. 25.

References

1. J Vasc Surg. 1998;27: 576-81.
2. J Vasc Surg. 2007; 45:328-34.
3. Semin Vasc Surg. 2000;13:No 1:10-19.
4. Minn Med. 2004:38-40.
5. Ann Thorac Surg. 2009;87:416-22.
6. Int J Angiol. 1999;8:87-90.
7. New techniques for thoracic outlet syndromes.
8. Ernesto Molina J. Springer. 2013.

Chapter 25
Extended Incision to Expose the Innominate Vein

In treating the syndrome of subclavian vein thrombosis after the first stage of the care was completed and the surgical intervention undertaken, most of the time the operation can be done as described in the previous Chap. 24. However occasionally after the first rib has been removed and the vein has been isolated and opened, the more proximal normal vein cannot be reached in order to place a widening patch into the normal wide open proximal or innominate vein because the incision stops at the sternum. The extension of the surgical incision can be undertaken without removing the clamps already placed on the vein. Everything is kept unchanged and without any additional risks an extension of the surgical field is implemented as described here.

Out of 249 patients operated for subclavian vein thrombosis, in 16% of them the more proximal normal subclavian vein could not be exposed in order to lay the vein patch appropriately beyond the fibrous obstruction. Therefore the subclavicular standard incision had to be extended medially across the sternum to reach the innominate vein. Here, it needs to be stressed that there is never a need to divide or remove the clavicle at any level to expose the subclavian or the innominate vein. The approach that is here presented is the safest acceptable route to expose both veins.

In this circumstance the skin incision is carried over the sternum to the midline (Fig. 25.1).The soft tissues are dissected off the manubrium of the sternum superiorly to expose the sternal notch. Using the cautery, the fibers and ligament across the notch are divided down to the bone level. This would allow to enter the mediastinum and digitally the retrosternal space is dissected from the top downwards. Now, also from the side laterally the soft tissue is dissected behind the sternum from the level where the rib was divided until this space connects with the dissection created from the top. This maneuver facilitates next to make a right-angle cut in the manubrium (Fig. 25.2).

The sternum is now split using a Neuroairtome. This instrument is preferred because the operator can make a right-angle turn while cutting the bone without stopping to arrange or change the direction of the incision. It is safer than using a

Fig. 25.1 An extension of
the surgical incision must
be made medially entering
the sternum as shown. *Scl*
Subclavian vein

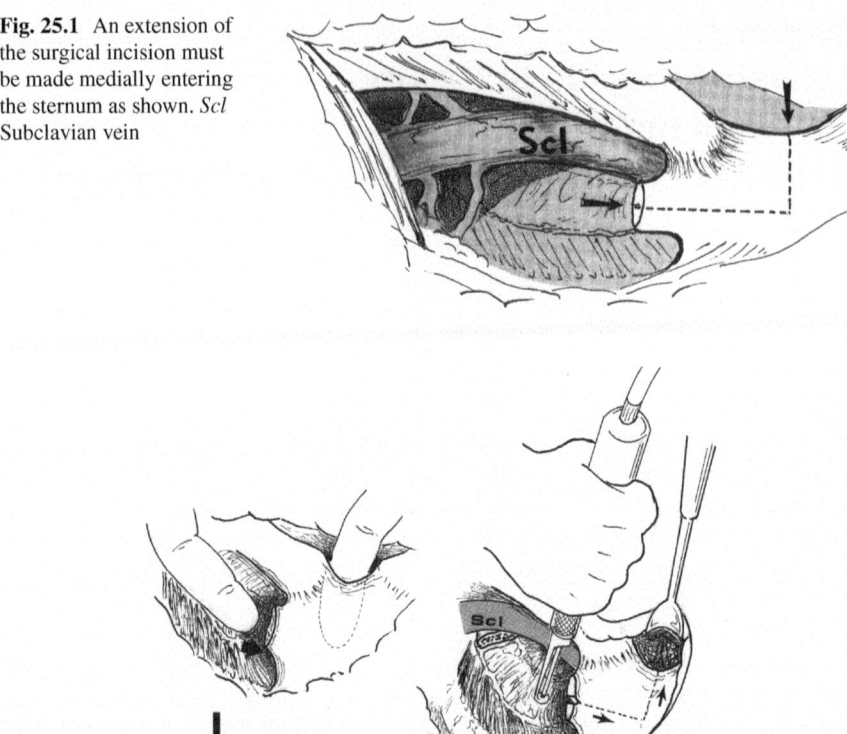

Fig. 25.2 The skin incision is carried over to the midline of the sternum. There is no need to make
a right-angle skin incision, just straight transverse. Using the cautery the sternal notch is dissected
and the retrosternal space is reached and with blunt dissection a finger can be passed downwards
to the level of the stump of the resected first rib. Laterally the dissection of the retrosternal space is
also carried out until the two spaces are connected. Using a Neuroairtome the manubrium of the
sternum is divided at right angle. *Scl* Subclavian vein

regular sternal saw. Once the sternum is divided, the upper separated fragment can
be retracted without interfering with the sternoclavicular joint (Fig. 25.3).

The vein is gently isolated and a vascular clamp can be applied in the normal
medial subclavian or in the innominate vein. During the dissection one must be
careful not to injure the phrenic nerve which should be separated from the vein
(Fig. 25.4). The previous venotomy done in the subclavian vein is now extended as
well until normal vein is found and the proper widening of the vein can be
accomplished.

After the vein stricture is corrected with the laid-on patch, the vascular clamps
are released and the chest incision can be closed.

To repair the sternum it is sufficient to do it with two heavy-wire sutures (gauge
6 or 8) as shown (Fig. 25.5), placed vertically and horizontally. To go through the

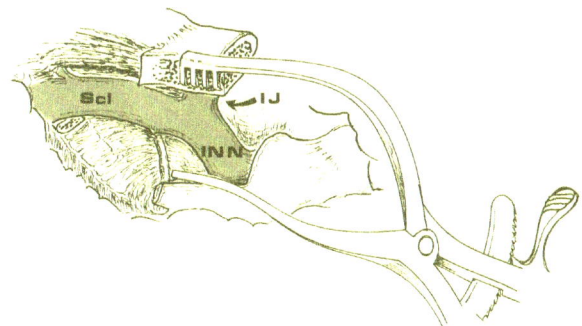

Fig. 25.3 The separated segment of sternum manubrium is retracted superiorly and the clavicular joint is left intact. Placing a mechanical retractor the entire area of the innominate vein is clearly exposed. With very gentle dissection the innominate vein is encircled and a vascular clamp can be applied. There is usually no need to divide the mammary vessels and one must be very careful of not injuring the phrenic nerve running medially. *INN* innominate, *Scl* subclavian vein, *IJ* internal jugular vein

Fig. 25.4 If necessary, occasionally, for control of the entire area, a vascular straight clamp may be placed at the base of the internal jugular vein. *Scl* subclavian vein, *INN* innominate vein, *IJ* internal jugular vein

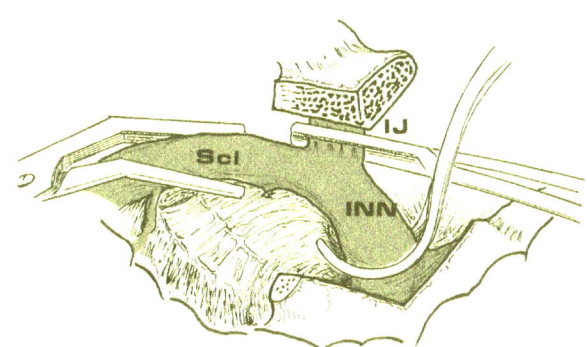

bone safely, a metal ribbon retractors should be placed under to protect the mediastinal organs (Figs. 25.6 and 25.7). It is preferable to make the holes with a drill rather than trying to forcefully press with the suture needles through the bone because in that maneuver the needle may not grab bone or slip causing unforeseen damage. The complete repair is shown (Fig. 25.8).

The routine postoperative anticoagulation regimen, as well as the need for venography, must be followed to verify the vein patency. As indicated in the previous chapter, the use of endovascular stent placement should be undertaken if residual stricture is present.

Restriction of physical activity must be strictly observed because if the repair falls apart, redoing it is not an easy task that will double the period of recovery. Therefore the wear of an arm sling is mandatory for a period of 8 weeks and no heavy type of exercise or activity is allowed for that period of time (Fig. 25.9).

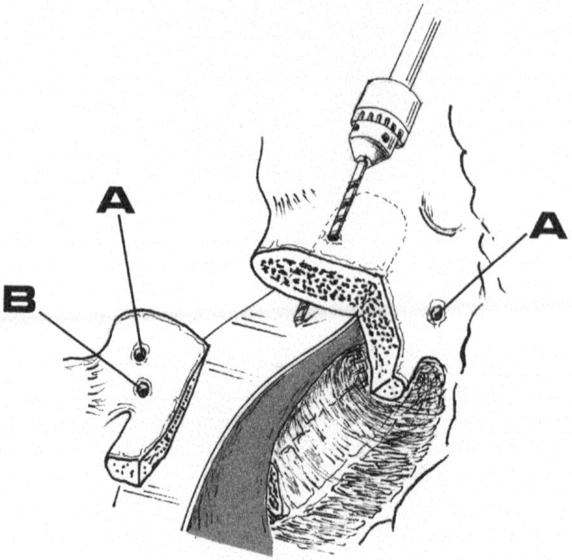

Fig. 25.5 To approximate
the sternal bone, only two
heavy-wire sutures are
necessary: one vertical and
the other horizontal. Make
sure that the stitches go
through bone and not soft
tissue

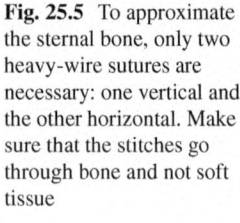

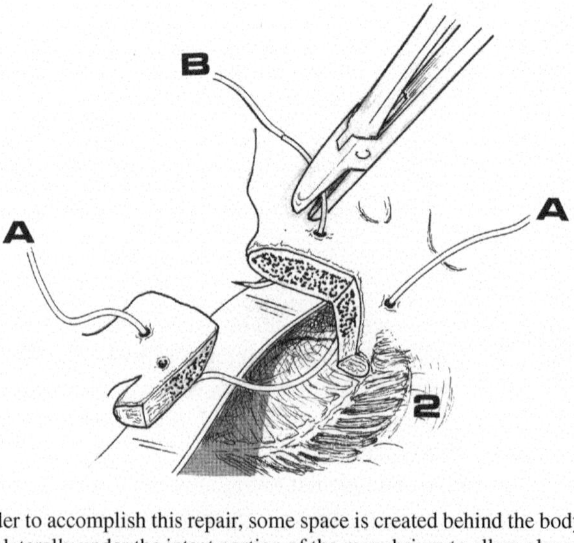

Fig. 25.6 In order to accomplish this repair, some space is created behind the body of the sternum
distally and also laterally under the intact portion of the manubrium to allow placement of the wire
sutures. A narrow type of ribbon retractor is placed behind the sternum to protect the mediastinal
organs. A standard drill is recommended to make the holes with and not to force the sharp needle
that comes with the suture. This will assure a smooth closure without causing any injury particularly when the sternum is strong and hard to penetrate

Fig. 25.7 Mediastinal
tissues are protected with a
ribbon retractor behind the
sternum

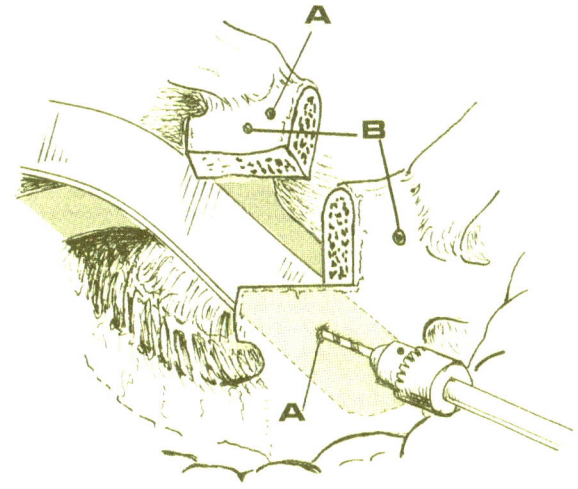

Fig. 25.8 This shows the
complete repair of the
incision and the vein patch
on the subclavian vein can
be seen in the background

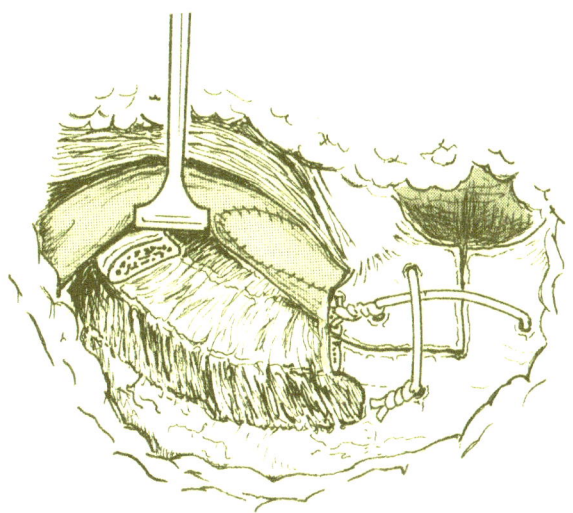

Fig. 25.9 The three stages of the operation. A small drain is placed in the wound. The pleural space is not entered. However if the pleura is violated, a chest tube drain must be placed to allow re-expansion of the lung

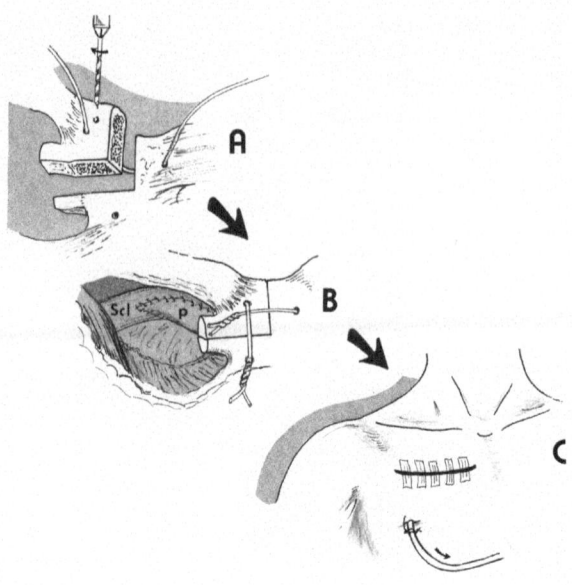

Reference

1. Semin Vasc Surg. 2000;13:10–19.

Chapter 26
Thoracic Outlet Syndromes Neurogenic and Arterial

There are three types of syndromes that involve compression or obstruction of the three structures that travel through the outlet of the chest, namely the brachial plexus, the subclavian artery, and the subclavian vein (Fig. 26.1). The latter of these three has been already described in the previous Chap. 25. The other two cannot be treated or operated with the same approach and require a different intervention.

Although the brachial plexus and the subclavian artery are running close together usually involved together, each one can be isolated involved without detectable abnormality in the function of the other. Frequently enough when the patient is

Fig. 26.1 Anatomy of the thoracic outlet. The first rib is shown with the anterior and posterior portions. The anterior contains the anterior scalene tendon which for this operation needs to be removed. Not so the subclavius tendon too far anterior which does not play any role in the compression of the brachial plexus or the subclavian artery. The posterior portion consists of the space through which the nerve and artery run and the medial scalene muscle that must be removed all the way back to the end of the rib at the joint with the vertebral transverse process

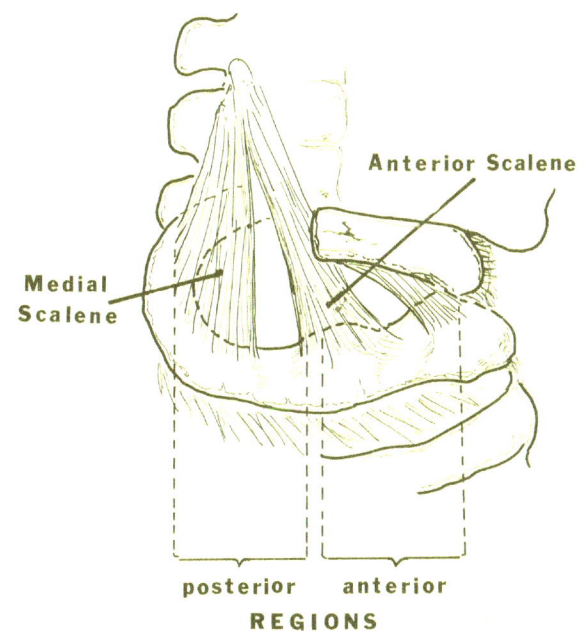

Anterior Scalene

Medial Scalene

posterior   anterior
REGIONS

© Springer International Publishing AG, part of Springer Nature 2018
J. E. Molina, *Cardiothoracic Surgical Procedures and Techniques*,
https://doi.org/10.1007/978-3-319-75892-3_26

tested for arterial compression and turns out negative, the patient is told that no compression is causing the symptoms and the patient is dismissed leaving it in a limbo. Neurogenic thoracic outlet compression is exclusively a clinical diagnosis which cannot be ruled out by any currently used laboratory tests. May be in the future with new advances in this area of health care some new methods more precise could be discovered or developed. However at present, only the clinical evaluation is available, which is nevertheless very reliable in experienced examiners.

Diagnosis

Persons suffering from these conditions are usually in the younger age group from teenagers to middle age, but it can occur also in older patients.

The patients usually complain of numbness or pain along the affected arm with maneuvers involving raising the arm over the head or even to the shoulder level. In women a common complaint is their inability to comb their hair or holding a hair dryer at the head level. As the symptoms become more severe, patients are even unable of driving their vehicles because they cannot maintain the hands at the steering wheel. In more severe cases if nothing is done atrophy of the hand and forearm muscles may gradually develop translated into weakness of the hand sometimes with inability of holding objects.

Several maneuvers implemented by the examining physicians usually establish the diagnosis. All these tests basically implement abduction of the arm to the shoulder level and over the head when the patient is sitting in an upright position. Within seconds the patient feels the pain radiating from the shoulder to the tip of the fingers. This is relieved by bringing the arm down. If compression of the subclavian artery is also present, the hand becomes pale and the radial pulse disappears. Some patients experience also dizziness and even nausea and vomiting in extreme cases.

Compression of the subclavian artery occurs in about 51% of the time observed with disappearance of the radial pulse. However the absence of this sign does not mean that compression is not occurring, particularly of the brachial plexus. The most reliable test in this situation is the performance of an ultrasound examination positioning the ultrasound probe over the subclavian zone while the patient elevates the affected arm. The position of the patient however must be sitting up straight and rising the arm over the head. The ultrasound technician should be trained in conducting this test properly to be interpreted by the radiologist. If the test is positive the treatment of choice is to proceed with decompression of the thoracic outlet.

The ultrasound exam is very important because in cases with chronic compression of the artery it may lead to the formation of a subclavian aneurysm with thrombus formation and peripheral embolization which has been documented in our institution. If the physician is unfamiliar with this complication and the patient is referred to physical therapy, in an attempt to avoid an operation, the ultrasound exam must always be done to prevent the occurrence of such serious complications.

The proper treatment for neurogenic or vascular thoracic outlet syndrome is surgical decompression. Physical therapy applied to relieve the symptoms usually is a temporary solution which often becomes an economic waste with no end in sight.

Although relief of the neurovascular compression can be performed implementing various surgical techniques, we recommend in our institution to do it using a dual approach. This means to make two incisions while the patient is positioned in a lateral decubitus while the affected arm is supported with a mechanical device attached to the operating table.

The key of success to achieve a total decompression of the thoracic outlet is the complete removal of the first rib which is often not achieved when its excision is attempted by making a single incision either in the axilla or in the supraclavicular area or using a subclavicular approach. The axillary incision alone does not provide adequate exposure to reach the posterior first rib insertion in the transverse process of the spine. The supraclavicular incision cannot reach the anterior portion of the rib because the clavicle is in the way. The subclavicular-only incision also prevents the exposure to the posterior end of the rib. The patient is left with an anterior and a posterior rib stump. The results of utilizing these approaches are persistence of the symptoms and recurrence of them that have to be treated with a reoperation with the obvious difficulties, risks, and unwillingness of any surgeon to undertake it.

Often enough operations using the trans-axillary-only approach remove only a small portion of the first rib and leave the both anterior and posterior ends in place. The reported failure of these operations is due to the incomplete removal of the rib and other muscular structures left intact and therefore incomplete decompression of the thoracic outlet. These known problems led us to the design the "DUAL APPROACH" implemented in our institution with excellent results reported in the literature.

The Operation

The operative procedure entails two stages which are conducted in the same session without changing the position of the patient in the operating table as explained below.

The first stage involves a subaxillary incision to expose the anterior half of the first rib (Fig. 26.2). After this is completed, and without closing the skin incision, the second stage follows with an incision in the back parallel to the trapezius muscle ridge. The patient is positioned in lateral decubitus with the affected arm suspended at right angle to the chest. In order to eliminate the need to have an assistant holding the arm in that position, an arm holder was devised that attaches to the operating table in the sterile operative field. This device is manufactured by Rultract Inc. of Cleveland, OH. It adequately holds the arm in the desired position. A pulley and crank can lift or lower the arm as needed during the dissection of the first rib. The pectoralis major muscle is retracted anteriorly and the latissimus dorsi muscle is retracted posteriorly. With the cautery the connective tissue is cleared off the rib and

Fig. 26.2 The axillary
incision allows to reach the
first rib and the muscular
tendons inserting in the
superior surface

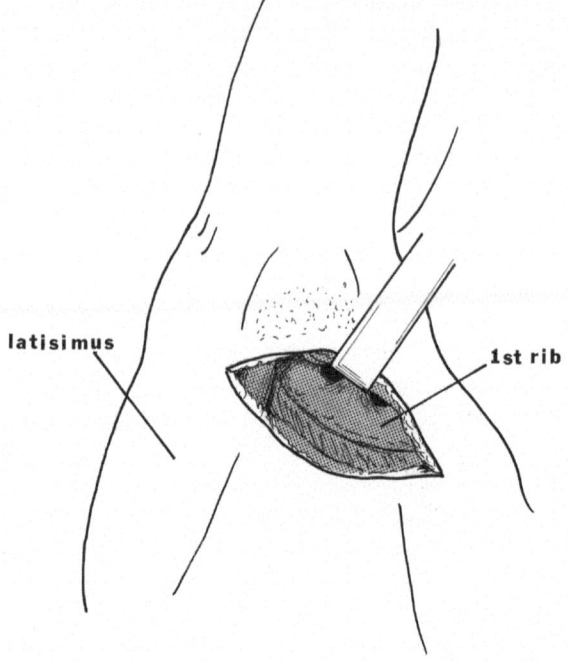

Fig. 26.3 Subperiosteal
dissection of the first rib
with a periosteal elevator

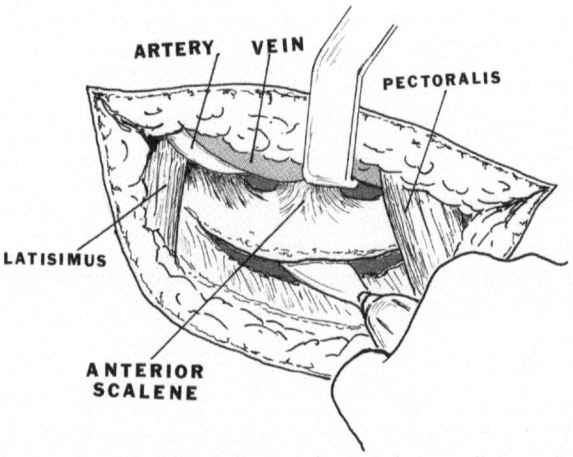

an incision is made in the inferior border to detach the periosteum (Fig. 26.3), until
sufficient space is created to digitally detach the pleura (Fig. 26.4). Retracting the
subclavian vein superiorly the tendon of the anterior scalene muscle is exposed,
isolated, and divided (Fig. 26.5). The superior border of the rib is cleared completely and some of the fibers of the medial scalene muscle can be divided (Fig. 26.6).
Once the rib is dissected free anteriorly it is divided but left in place. The incision is

Fig. 26.4 Digital
dissection is gently done to
detach the pleura off the
rib in its entire exposed
length

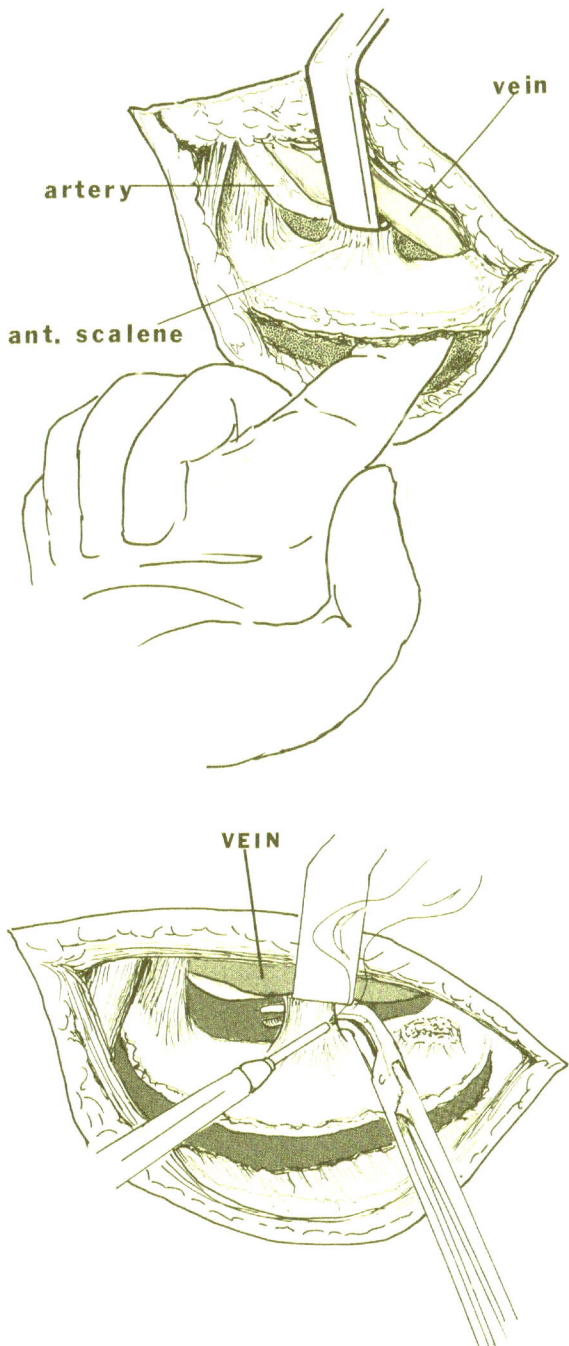

Fig. 26.5 The anterior
scalene tendon is now
safely divided while the
subclavian vein is retracted
superiorly

Fig. 26.6 The rib is now
divided at its anterior end.
This completes the first
stage of the operation

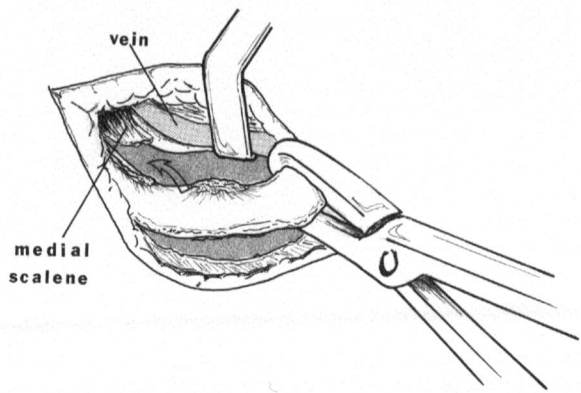

packed with a sponge soaked in antibiotic solution. The arm of the patient is taken off the arm holder and placed along the patient body. The stage one is now complete and we direct the attention to undertake the second stage.

Second stage. Without changing the position of the patient, an incision is made in the back parallel to the trapezius ridge from the spine toward the shoulder (Fig. 26.7). As the trapezius muscle is encountered, the fibers are separated in their direction but not divided. In the next plane the first muscle encountered is the levator of the scapula which is also retracted laterally toward the shoulder (Fig. 26.8). Careful dissection is done to prevent any damage to the nerve which would cause a winged scapula syndrome postoperatively. The first rib is now exposed. The superior border is dissected with the cautery detaching the fibers of the medial scalene muscle all the way toward the spine until the joint to the spine transverse process is reached. Usually the posterior scalene muscle that inserts on the second rib does not need to be divided but only retracted unless it is obstructing the exposure. Now the inferior border of the rib is incised detaching the intercostal muscle to the second rib. Digital maneuver helps to let the pleura fall away from the rib and creates sufficient space to proceed with division of the rib at the junction with the spine (Fig. 26.9). The rib is now removed from the field. The incision is closed in a routine manner all the way to the skin level.

We now return to the subaxillary incision that was left open and we proceed to close it. A drain is placed in the extrapleural space previously occupied by the removed rib and the skin incision is closed in the preferred manner. This completes the operation to decompress the thoracic outlet.

Fig. 26.7 After the first stage of this operation is done, the arm of the patient is removed from the mechanical arm holder and laid along the patient's chest. A second incision is made posteriorly parallel to the trapezius ridge

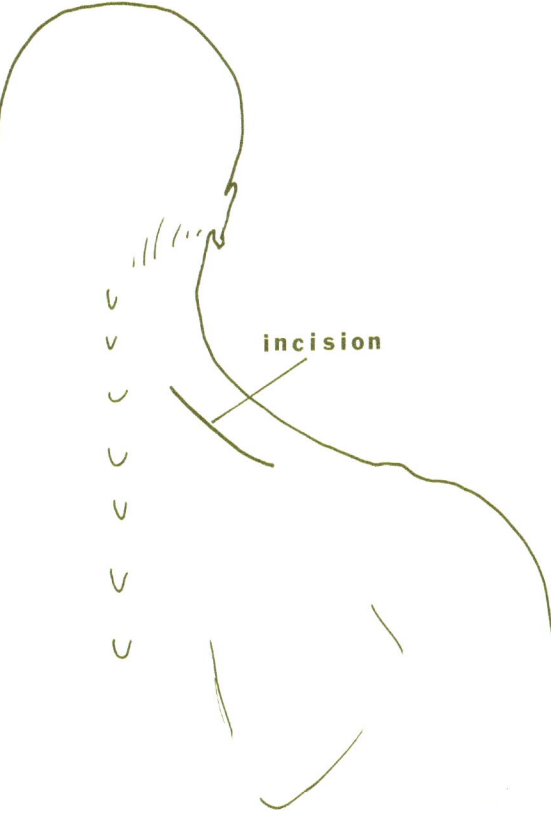

incision

Fig. 26.8 The fibers of the trapezius muscle are split in their anatomical direction but should not be divided. The muscle levator of the scapula is retracted anteriorly. The medial scalene muscle is divided detaching it from the superior aspect of the first rib. The posterior scalene muscle that inserts on the second rib is left intact

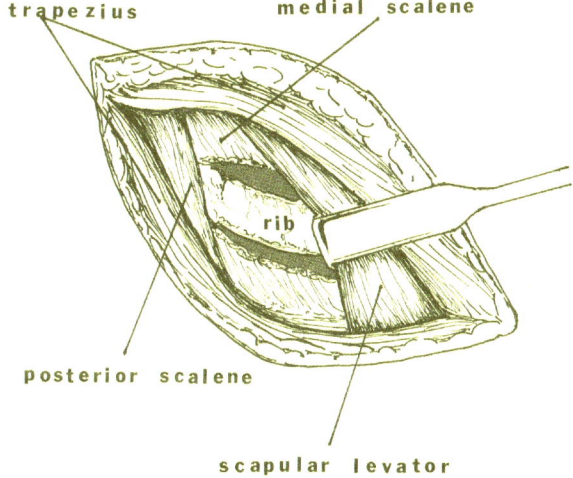

trapezius medial scalene

rib

posterior scalene

scapular levator

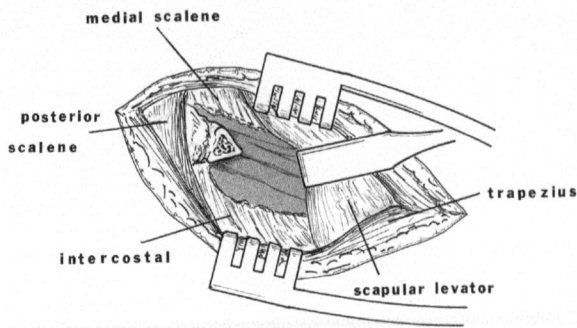

Fig. 26.9 Once the first rib is completely isolated, it is divided and removed from the field. The level at which it is divided is at the joint with the transverse vertebral process. This will assure total decompression of the nerve and the artery, and no recurrence of the patient's symptoms. The trunks of the brachial plexus are often clearly visualized at the bottom of the incision

Reference

1.   J Am Coll Surg. 1998;187:39–45.

Index

© Springer International Publishing AG, part of Springer Nature 2018
J. E. Molina, *Cardiothoracic Surgical Procedures and Techniques*,
https://doi.org/10.1007/978-3-319-75892-3

The manufacturer's authorised representative in the EU is Springer
Nature Customer Service Centre GmbH, Europaplatz 3, 69115 Heidelberg,
Germany. If you have any concerns regarding our products, please
contact ProductSafety@springernature.com

Printed and bound by CPI Group (UK) Ltd, Croydon, CR0 4YY
29/04/2026
02099451-0016